Praise for *Your Better Instincts*

"Deeply considered and personal, Dr. Stacy Irvine's book is one of the most contemplative I've ever read about health and instinct, and how we can be our best selves by being ourselves."

DAVE BIDINI author and musician

"*Your Better Instincts* takes an idea that is as old as time and makes it new, relevant and actionable for today. This book feels like a conversation with a trusted, wise and (very) fun friend who is gently reminding us how to lead a life well lived."

BRUCE SELLERY money columnist, CBC Radio and *Cityline*

"A fascinating voyage into the human psyche that puts words to the things we cannot see but that move us nonetheless."

DR. DEBORAH MACNAMARA author of *Rest, Play, Grow* and clinical counsellor

"*Your Better Instincts* will help you turn off the noise out there and tune in to the wisdom inside yourself. Dr. Stacy Irvine is a sage for anyone who wants to live their best life. This book will teach you to trust yourself and find your inner confidence."

LYNDA REEVES founder, *House & Home* magazine

"*Your Better Instincts* explores an ancient concept—instinct—with a unique perspective. It allows us to better understand how we can thrive in and contribute to our planet in a positive way. When we realize that these instinctual pathways are designed with purpose, it becomes easier to find our own happiness within the journey."

DAVE SALMONI animal trainer, television personality and producer

YOUR
BETTER
INSTINCTS

YOUR BETTER INSTINCTS

UNCOVER YOUR INNER POWER
to IMPROVE HEALTH, HAPPINESS
and PERFORMANCE

Dr. STACY IRVINE

PAGE TWO

Cataloguing in publication information is available
from Library and Archives Canada.
ISBN 978-1-989603-62-8 (hardcover)
ISBN 978-1-989603-63-5 (ebook)

Page Two
pagetwo.com

Edited by Amanda Lewis
Copyedited by John Sweet
Proofread by Alison Strobel
Cover and interior design by Taysia Louie
Author photos by David Perry
Printed and bound in Canada by Friesens
Distributed in Canada by Raincoast Books
Distributed in the US and internationally
by Macmillan

21 22 23 24 25   5 4 3 2 1

yourbetterinstincts.com

AS A PERSON who relies on her instincts, I would like to dedicate this book to my family... who could rightfully argue I may rely on them too much. Also, my patients and clients, and the athletes I have coached over the years. You have had to endure way more than a "normal" amount of my enthusiastic ideas, opinions and theories on too many things to count!

I would also like to acknowledge and thank my parents, Sharon and Dale Fyke, for instilling in me the confidence to trust my inner powers and strengths. This confidence allowed me to enter any arena, observe, learn from and sometimes even compete with the best, while embracing both the failures and the wins.

Finally, to all the nature explorers and animal lovers out there, I hope you will enjoy reading this book as much as I enjoyed writing it!

CONTENTS

INTRODUCTION
Time to Alter Our Course

I AM WRITING THIS introduction as we begin our seventh week of isolation during the COVID-19 pandemic. I hope I am not stirring up horrible memories for you. In Canada, it seems we have weathered this life-changing event fairly well so far, while some countries have experienced devastating death tolls along with massive economic turmoil.

Totum Life Science, a health and sports medicine business that I co-own with my husband, has been closed for the duration of this time. Our lives, as well as the lives of our many employees, have been thrust into a stressful waiting game. We have no idea when it will be safe to reopen, or what that will look or feel like. Even in just the first few weeks, the number of small business closures in our neighbourhood was shocking. Our time in isolation has been one of extreme stress, with lots of tears and emotional outbursts. We do our best to contain these expressions within the walls of our house. Our three children are all too aware of what is happening because our home is now our office, and the continued conversations with the bank and landlords can be heard by all.

Together, the world has celebrated birthdays, weddings and even Earth Day in isolation. I mention Earth Day because the repeated narrative that day was something along this theme:

We were warned that a pandemic was coming, and we did nothing to change our way of life. Today we are suffering the consequences.

We have also been warned for many years that climate change will destroy our planet. After surviving this pandemic, will we continue to ignore these warnings about our environment? Or will we decide to make some difficult changes and find a different path?

Along with the pandemic, we experienced a rise in race-related and Black Lives Matter protests in response to the murder of George Floyd. There have been many lessons learned from our time in isolation, along with a constant streaming of videos, jokes, TikTok dances and protest chants that are constantly sent to our inboxes and social media feeds. One video that went viral early on was called *The Great Realisation*, a poem (now book) by Tomos Roberts that was read as a bedtime story. This poem was set in a time post pandemic, and it described how humanity learned to appreciate what was important and improved ourselves and our future as a result. Many of us can relate to Roberts's inspiring words, and I was amazed at how much the sentiment was familiar and inspiring to me as I was writing this book. Here are a few lines that particularly resonated with me.

It was a world of waste and wonder, of poverty and plenty.

We noticed families had stopped talking. That's not to say they never spoke. But the meaning must have melted and the work-life balance broke.

And the children's eyes grew squarer, and every toddler had a phone.

We'd forgotten how to run. We swapped the grass for tarmac. Shrunk the parks until there were none.

The tone of the poem then changes to describe how, because of our time in isolation, we slowly began to change: "sometimes you get sick... before you start feeling better" and your "old habits became extinct."

One of the lines actually got me to stand right up out of my chair almost cheering (also because, during this time, I found myself sitting *way* too much on Zoom meetings, conference calls and so on, so I embraced any excuse to stand and move):

> But while we were all hidden, amidst the fear... We dusted off our instincts. We remembered how to smile.

I felt as though Roberts was talking directly to me! How did he know I was busy toiling away at this book, trying to find a good way to explain to everyone how important our instincts are to our ability to thrive in life?

This simple, brilliant line and the concept of "dust[ing] off our instincts" captures exactly what I hope this book can be for everyone. Our instincts are a part of us and always have been. Over the last couple of centuries, much of humanity has created structures and systems that allow us to ignore our instincts, and not even attempt to develop them to their full potential. The goal of this book is to help you understand how important it is to honour your basic human instincts—for the sake of your health, your performance and ultimately your happiness. Your instincts will serve you through good times, bad times and even pandemic times.

When I began writing this book, a pandemic was a phenomenon I had studied in university, and something I was vaguely aware had happened over a century ago. We have all been completely re-educated on what constitutes a pandemic—and if you are reading this book, you have survived what is probably your first one. As we were learning and trying to survive, we were also bombarded by media explaining our chances of survival and why COVID-19 has proven to be so lethal. Even as the first cases emerged, writers and personalities were emphatically stressing that our current lifestyle needs to change if we are going to "win this war." At the time of printing this book, we are approaching 170 million cases and 3.5 million deaths globally.

That does not feel like a win to me, but in a big effort to learn from our mistakes I have found it important to apply the data against the basic human instincts we will explore in this book. There are many clear variables that we now understand drastically increase our vulnerability and susceptibility to illness as a population:

- Living in crowded urban centres where physical distancing is difficult and the lack of space makes active lifestyles a challenge

- Living in extreme poverty with limited access to hygienic waste management, food distribution and clean drinking water

- Animals being slaughtered for food on a massive scale while living in extremely crowded environments

- Caring for our elderly by placing them in long-term care homes that are sometimes not well equipped to deliver an optimal quality of life, and in some sad cases even feature inhumane living conditions

- Overcrowded and understaffed jails, often found in countries where private companies profit from incarceration, and strategies to fill these facilities and prolong the periods of jail time while paying little attention to rehabilitation and social support systems that are needed to prevent crime

- Living in a greed-obsessed, materialistic culture where many are one paycheque away from homelessness or even bankruptcy

- Having no ability to obtain food or water that does not come from a grocery store or a municipal water supply

- Being drastically immunocompromised because of lifestyle choices such as smoking, obesity and/or drug/alcohol addiction

- Having a decreased ability to handle stressful situations because of poor lifestyle choices, including insufficient sleep, inadequate nutrition, lack of exercise and/or shortage of meaningful human connections

In many ways, this pandemic highlighted some of our weaknesses as a society, but it also tested our strength and resilience. Some citizens were further divided because of poor leadership and mixed messages, while others were brought closer together as they sacrificed personal wants to accelerate the common good of their communities. We found heroes within the ranks of our health care providers and scientists. We also learned that although we may feel we live our lives in similar ways, the challenges we face in tough times are often determined by our specific situation.

I hope that the personal stories and case studies in the following chapters will help you better understand your own instincts and behaviours. It is my strongest desire to provide you with information that will enhance your life in the best way possible. I include examples of things I have learned from the athletes I coach and the patients I treat, as well as lessons derived from my own experiences, to help you understand how powerful our instincts really are. I interviewed several "high-performers" for Part Two, and I selected these particular people because their expertise is causally related to the instincts we will be exploring. Hopefully, you will use this book to find practical ways to harness your instincts and unleash this "superpower" that has been a part of us since... well, forever!

To Help Us Organize Our Thoughts

Writing about a topic such as instincts can be challenging, as you will see in the following chapters. Our personal beliefs about our instincts can vary, and understanding how they affect each aspect of our life can add to this confusion. As we dive into the topic, there may be moments where you wonder, "What is she talking about?!" or "Why is this part even in here?" I hope this book enhances your curiosity and inspires many more questions about *your own* instincts and how they relate to *your* personal experiences.

I have identified three main groups of instincts: **instincts for health**, **instincts for performance** and **instincts for happiness** (see the table on page 216). Obviously, there will be some overlap as we meander through these pages of research, scientific theories, personal stories and expert opinions.

PART ONE

UNLOCKING THE POWER OF YOUR INSTINCTS

1

Why Instincts?

It is not the strongest of the species that survives, nor the most intelligent that survives, it is the one that is the most adaptable to change. The very essence of instinct, is that it is followed independently of reason.

CHARLES DARWIN

W HEN WE ARE born, we are thrust into society, completely dependent on others for our survival. Our parents or possibly other caregivers provide us with the necessities of life, and we begin our journey toward being a fully developed, independent person. Our genetic makeup is determined by the generations of relatives who have come before us, and it then becomes our responsibility to do what we can with the attributes we inherit. Centuries of research has shown that how we develop and grow as human beings is within our control. We can determine how strong we are, how fast we are, how coordinated we are and many other things within our genetic limits and environmental opportunities. It would seem logical that every human being would have a desire to optimize this potential when presented with the opportunity to do so.

This concept is certainly not a new or original way of thinking, as the critically acclaimed 18th-century novelist Jean Paul wrote many centuries ago: "To make as much out of oneself as could be made out of the stuff."

Our human instincts are some of the strongest influencers of our health and survival. When we design or adopt a lifestyle that ignores our basic instincts or even simply fails to understand and acknowledge them, we suffer as a species. We can find supporting examples of this neglect from other species in all forms of nature and wildlife:

animals living in zoos, whales living in captivity, animals mass-produced and slaughtered for food, pesticides sprayed abundantly on our fields and even the vast amounts of plastic containers contaminating our oceans and water supply. In so many cases, we have ignored our basic instincts and replaced them with the rewards of convenience and the feeling of instant gratification. We are now learning, through many difficult situations, including death in some cases, that this is probably not the best way to exist on this planet.

Our species has moved rapidly through various phases of agricultural advancement followed by an age of industry, and we are now entering an era dominated by technology. At the same time, there are indications that many of us may not be living our lives in the best way possible. According to the Government of Canada's statistics for 2018, the average life expectancy in Canada is 80 years for males and 84 years for females. According to similar data from 2011, the life expectancy of Indigenous males is 70.5 and for females it is 77 (although these data are difficult to interpret because of the lack of birth and death reports on many reserves). The infant mortality rate is reported as being twice as high for Indigenous populations compared with non-Indigenous populations. These numbers are incredible when you think that, in many cases, Indigenous and non-Indigenous people are born and live in the same communities. All human beings have comparable instincts. Indigenous populations have similar genetic origins as the European colonizers who arrived after them. Why, then, should their life expectancy be so much lower than that of the general population? If you have ever spent time on a reserve, or even gained a historical understanding of the many hardships Indigenous peoples have endured over this past century, you will probably understand part of the answer to this question.

In the United States, life expectancy has declined over the last few years. Overall, our North American population is suffering more from what are called "diseases of despair," leading to many more deaths from suicide and drug overdose. Rates of obesity and its associated metabolic disorders, such as diabetes, are still rising and unfortunately affecting even younger populations. Our younger populations also have a much higher diagnosis rate for depression and attention deficit hyperactivity disorder (ADHD). Over the past few years in Canada, experts have given our youth a mark of D when it comes to their current levels of activity and exercise.

At the same time, medical and health science advances over this past century have been breathtaking, and they show no signs of slowing down. We have made incredible progress in our understanding of nutritional science, cardiovascular health and how to improve human performance. Most of this information is available to anyone with access to the Internet. So we must ask, if the basic answers to how we can lead incredibly healthy lives are available to us whenever we need them, why do we not act upon this information every single day? For some reason, simply having the information does not seem to be enough. We need to gain a better understanding of the barriers to personal healthy habits, or possibly discover what is demotivating or distracting the majority of our populations.

With respect to life in more recent times, I find it interesting that we can be constantly, and often instantly, connected to people all over the world and yet, at the same time, "extreme loneliness" related to a "growing incidence of depression" regularly makes the headlines. How can this be? Perhaps we have not yet found a harmonious way to exist within supportive communities in this technology-driven world.

Although evolutionary scientists are not in complete agreement about this, *Homo sapiens* as a species inhabited Earth approximately 200,000 years ago. Prior to this time, other versions of our first human ancestors appeared, about 5 to 7 million years ago. The bodies and brains we walk around with today are not drastically different from those of the first *Homo sapiens*; however, our lifestyle, movement patterns and diet could not be more different.

Our instincts represent
efficient pathways
designed to enhance
most of our regular
everyday functions.

———————

However, there are small pockets of our global population that are exceeding the norms when compared with some of the more industrialized hubs of the world. Life expectancy in certain countries is remarkable, along with awesome feats in human performance and even lifelong happiness. Why are these benefits experienced by only a few and not by our populations as a whole? If we can gain a better understanding of our basic human instincts and how they drive certain behaviours, we can learn to use agriculture and technology to enhance our health, to help us perform better in the undertakings that inspire us, and to increase our happiness.

Each of our instincts has a specific role to play in our overall development, along with our daily habits and routines. It may be helpful to think of this system as an embedded circuitry with which we are born. When we ignore the intended functions of this circuitry, we can easily run into problems. Likewise, you would not use your toaster to make a delicious fruit smoothie because you understand that a toaster is "built" and "wired" for a completely different function. A more subtle analogy would be arguing with an audiophile that they can just as well listen to music from their computer speakers rather than playing albums on their expensive turntable and sound system. When we ignore the basic plan and fundamental purpose of something, or when we do not understand how to use a particular technology in the right way, we are failing to realize its potential. The human body is a masterful design involving millions of cell interactions, many of which we do not yet fully understand. Our instincts represent efficient pathways designed to enhance most of our regular everyday functions.

Instincts influence almost all aspects of our lives, including our conscious actions and unconscious behaviours. Our instincts have been with us for as long as we have been a species, and some patterns are present even before birth. Instincts are like a human superpower that we might often ignore because we do not need to pay attention to them for them to do an excellent job. Instincts help us survive, they help us stay healthy, they help us perform better, often without us even recognizing that they are working for us.

TRAINING TOOL: Why We Should Understand Our Instincts

If we recognize instincts as pathways throughout our bodies and brains that are already partially formed, in order to enhance our performance or health, and perhaps even our happiness, it is most efficient to follow a path that is already there. For example, picture yourself standing at the edge of a beautiful ancient forest. There are huge tree trunks in every direction, and the forest floor is covered with a thick bed of ferns. There is a visible path through the forest, a creek running on one side of you, and you were told that there are steep ravine drop-offs and edges throughout the forest. A smart, experienced hiker would take the path already formed in front of them to make their way through the forest, because they know that this path is there for a reason. It is the most efficient and safe way to travel through this area. Some people may choose to ignore the path and venture out in a different direction, through the bushes or navigating the creek. They will have a different experience, and one that is probably less efficient and more dangerous than that of the hikers who chose the path that was already formed.

If we ignore our instinctual patterns, we force our bodies to carve out new pathways, and some of these diversions can have negative consequences. Our human bodies were originally designed to move regularly and then rest between movements. When we ignore the idea of regular movement, for instance by prolonged sitting or becoming too sedentary, our physical health suffers, along with our mental capacity. Many of us have chosen lifestyles where we are sitting for the majority of the day, even though that is not how we were designed to exist—sort of like using a toaster to make a smoothie. If we keep trying to force a toaster to make a smoothie, we will probably suffer some negative outcomes. When talking about our instincts, following the path of least resistance is not always a bad thing.

RECOMMENDED READING: *The Blue Zones of Happiness: Lessons from the World's Happiest People* by Dan Buettner

2

How Our Instincts Motivate Us

My instincts never fail me,
But I fail them all the time...

SISSY GAVRILAKI

HUMANS' DIFFERING MOTIVATIONS have always fascinated me. During a basic first-year course in kinesiology at the University of Saskatchewan, I remember learning that 30 percent of our North American population will want to exercise and train hard, just because that is what they are genetically designed to do. At that particular time in my life, I was one of those who was exercising and training hard, so I assumed I was part of this 30 percent, and so were the people I worked with who liked exercise. The other 70 percent were extremely difficult to motivate, I thought, and that was basically the end of the story.

I loved studying kinesiology and all things related to training, physiology and the human body. As a competitive heptathlete, I believed that my understanding of the science behind the training would give me an edge over my competitors. I am not sure if my studies ever had a real impact on my personal performance, but it was a perfect environment for learning and retaining vast amounts of information. Many of the ideas I would hear about in lectures, or the muscle systems I would be dissecting in anatomy, would be right there in front of me at practice at the end of the day. Add to this the fact that I was not the most naturally talented athlete; I managed to keep up through tons of hard work and extra practice. The systems and research I digested in my daily lectures had very real applications in my actual life and in the development of my training programs at that time. It was an ideal learning environment.

After graduating from kinesiology, I went on to finish a master's degree in exercise physiology. I was still training as an athlete, but now I was also working regularly as a coach. At the same time, research in exercise science was progressing rapidly, and it was significantly changing the way we trained, ate and even recovered. I soon realized, as I encountered challenges with some of the groups I was coaching, that the 30 percent rule did not exactly explain everything. More importantly, this idea was useless when you are trying to make actual improvements in human performance or motivate someone to work harder or attempt a difficult skill using a new technique. Having the genetics to move well and to be faster, stronger or more powerful than most humans is one part of success, but equally important is the motivation and intellectual capacity to use those skills in the best way possible.

My main event in track and field was the heptathlon; you participate in seven track events and score points in each, and the athlete with the highest score at the end of two days of competing wins. Because of my training for the heptathlon, along with my university studies and research, I was well experienced to coach throws, jumps and sprints. I cared deeply about all the athletes I was working with and used every bit of information I could find to increase their success. At the same time, I was asked to help coach the university football team during their off-season to improve their running techniques and hopefully enhance their strength and speed. The University of Saskatchewan had a fantastic football program at that time and would go on to win many Vanier Cup championships. It was phenomenally exciting to be working with this group of talented athletes, many of whom are still close friends today.

A comment I would hear occasionally from the football coaches, referring to one of the players, was "He has all the tools, but he is missing the tool box!" It took me a while to figure out what they meant. Part of my coaching job involved testing the players in various aspects of speed, agility, power and strength. Some of these tests would be similar to what you find in today's NFL Combine. For those unfamiliar with it, the NFL Combine is a series of athletic events used as a standardized way to evaluate players prior to the draft. Similarly, we were often interested in how fast players could run 40 metres, for example, and we would continue to test this as their training progressed. However, while certain players would have spectacular performances at the track, this did not always translate to the field. I would excitedly present some of these amazing results to the coaches, and the statement about the tool box would be repeated to me. What they meant was that even though the player was incredibly physically talented, he could not translate that talent into game-day performance.

I started to think about motivation and intellectual capacity again. In retrospect, if I had wanted to predict which freshmen players in that group would have the most success in football, I would have been way more accurate if I had evaluated their levels of motivation, their work behaviours and habits, and their ability to tap into their basic instincts for the game of football. While the pure raw talent that shows up as a result of our genetic abilities is a significant part of the picture, it is probably not the most important contributor to overall success in a game or a real-life situational environment.

Motivation Is Important for All High-Performers

Fast-forward a few years and I have moved from Saskatoon to Winnipeg. I am taking a "break" from my studies following the completion of my master's degree, to train and teach with Canada's Royal Winnipeg Ballet. I had left behind the world of science-focused training and moved into a realm of historical, artistic and authoritative

While the pure raw talent
that shows up as a result
of our genetic abilities is a
significant part of the picture,
it is probably not the
most important contributor
to overall success.

———————

instruction, directed at some of the best ballet performers in the world. This style—which demanded sacrifice, discipline and emotional investment—also resulted in the performers' exhaustion, explosive behaviours, and the blood, sweat and tears that often surface from that level of commitment. I was privileged to have an intimate view of these training techniques for three years working within this exceptional program. These performers did not worry only about their strength, flexibility and endurance, but also about how they connected with their audience emotionally and what they looked like onstage from an aesthetic point of view. It was an incredible learning experience.

After a few years in Winnipeg, I felt it was time to get back to academics. Tim, my boyfriend at the time, was also finishing his master's degree in biomechanics. We decided to move to Toronto because it would be a good place to pursue our Ph.D.s, with many potential universities within a few hours of each other. We both began teaching positions at the University of Toronto and I also started working as a kinesiologist and personal trainer at the Toronto Athletic Club. Working with a population in Toronto that mainly consisted of downtown Bay Street types, this was my first exposure to a more "regular" population as opposed to elite athletes, and motivation levels differed. How could I get a busy mom with two young children and a stressful job as an investment banker to take the 20 minutes required daily to do her boring rehab exercises to prevent her neck pain? How could I persuade my Type A CEO workaholic party animal to get enough sleep so that he would benefit from his training sessions and not be constantly injured?

During these years working with clients and patients, I realized that instead of doing a Ph.D., I should probably look for more education and training related to rehabilitation and diagnosis of orthopaedic injuries. I applied to the Ontario Chiropractic College in Toronto and was accepted. That education consumed my next four years, although I somehow managed to keep working within our brand new and rapidly growing business, Totum Life Science. After working for a few years in the fitness and health industry in Toronto, Tim and I had decided to branch out and start our own business. This was not without extreme challenges, as two science-trained "jocks" tried their best to navigate a whole new world of business in a city where we basically knew no one.

In 2004, I graduated with a doctorate in chiropractic, and one month after graduation I gave birth to our first child. During my doctorate, I was required to retake all of the hard sciences I had studied many years earlier—biochemistry, anatomy, physiology and neuro-anatomy, to name a few—in addition to more practical training in radiology, nutrition and orthopaedic assessment. It was an exhausting and often very stressful time, simply because of the volume of memorization required, but I earned that degree feeling I had covered enough material to be a significant contributor to the world of health care and athletic training.

One thing, though, was missing: I did not receive any formal education explaining personal motivation and human behaviour, although I was observing it and being challenged by it every day. Once I finished my final board exams and returned to seeing patients, coaching athletes and training clients, I again felt that a better understanding of human behaviour would be critically important to the results I was trying to find for my patients and clients. All the physiological and anatomical information in the world would not lead to exceptional results if I was not able to effectively transfer this knowledge and find ways to motivate people.

Fast-forward approximately 20 years and my now-husband and I are still working hard, running Totum Life Science, with over 100 team members and five locations in Toronto. Totum comprises a fantastic group of highly dedicated professionals who manage to impress and inspire us every single day, along with an outstanding group of patients, clients and athletes who include some of Canada's top business leaders, professional athletes and even some celebrities. I am thrilled to say that my time at Totum never feels like work.

Over the past 30 years, I have seen many changes in how we treat patients, train athletes and even book appointments or use technology to improve the efficiency of the care we deliver. The digital advances in health care have been remarkable, with things like electronic medical records, virtual health delivery, along with assessment and testing tools that allow for faster and more accurate diagnosis of many conditions. Once artificial intelligence, quantum computing and machine learning are more involved in this field, I am sure we will experience incredible progress related to our understanding and optimization of human health. In that same period, however, I cannot say I have seen drastic improvements in the overall health of our society. We have some amazing outliers in the areas of human performance and longevity. There are a select few regions of the planet that have increased life expectancy, and our athletes continue to run faster, throw farther and grow stronger, but we also have dismal rates of obesity, cardiovascular disease, cancer and mental health issues.

We often talk about the concept of *willpower* when we are attempting to improve our overall health and the habits that impact our health. We view healthy and successful people as those who have tons of willpower, which enables them to always do the right thing and make good choices. We feel bad about ourselves and sometimes disappointed if we cannot maintain the level of discipline required to achieve our goals of losing weight, being more present or even exercising. But when we are living a lifestyle that causes us to be regularly exhausted and stressed out, our willpower can easily be defeated. This is where our instincts come in. As our willpower diminishes, our instincts can and will take over if we let them.

TRAINING TOOL: Instincts and Motivation

If our lives were designed in a way that respected and aligned with our basic instincts, we would find an easier path to health and happiness. We would also require less willpower to avoid negative habits, because our subconscious mind would be leading us in a better direction—even when we were tired or stressed out. If you often feel as though you do not reach your goals owing to a lack of willpower, look more into the structure of your life surrounding those goals. Can you change this structure so that you do not need to rely on your willpower so much?

For example, if we know that our bodies instinctually like to be in regular motion, we should look for opportunities to place regular "movement snacks" into our day. These are not workouts, but things like walking to work, taking the stairs at lunch or walking to a bathroom that is farther away when we are taking a break. Because this is how our bodies were instinctually designed to behave, it improves both our chemistry and physiology, making us feel better both mentally and physically.

Adequate rest is extremely important when it comes to our ability to motivate ourselves. We always tell our young athletes that a good training session starts the night before, with at least eight hours of sleep. Doing your best to improve your sleep environment, by removing the things that can interfere with it, such as screens, alcohol or even inconsistent sleep patterns, can have a major positive impact on your ability to maintain a high level of motivation.

Finally, we need to accept that many aspects of our lives might shift in ways we cannot control. The 2020 pandemic is a perfect example of this. We had learned to live, eat, shop, socialize and even exercise in certain habitual ways. Suddenly these things were drastically altered, and we had to adapt to a new way of life. Across the world we heard stories of depression and mental health issues, which affect motivation and willpower. The important thing to remember is that your struggle can be caused by external factors, and if this is the case, there is no point dwelling on your circumstances and your inability to be motivated. Accurate assessment and adaptation are the keys to finding your new strategies for motivation and willpower.

RECOMMENDED READING: *Mindset: The New Psychology of Success* by Carol S. Dweck

3

Understanding Our Instincts

My mind empties,
my heart opens, my spirit soars.

RICHARD WAGAMESE,
EMBERS

THERE IS A well-supported theory in psychology that we probably have our most brilliant thoughts when our mind is empty, when we are not actively trying to figure something out, or when we are engaged in a familiar task such as showering, driving or even mowing the lawn. The nub of the idea is that our subconscious mind, where our instincts live, has an almost instant processing and executing system when compared with the speed and effectiveness of the conscious or cognitive processing pathways in our brain. Malcolm Gladwell talks extensively about this concept in his book *Blink: The Power of Thinking without Thinking*. I wish that during my years as a competitive athlete I had understood the insights that *Blink* provides. At the end of the book, Gladwell writes: "It is not enough simply to explore the hidden recesses of our unconscious. Once we know how the mind works—and about the strengths and weaknesses of human judgement—it is our responsibility to act."

I agree with Gladwell's insights into this complex world of neurophysiology. When we understand how the mind works, we have a responsibility to act, especially those of us working in the fields of health and human performance—along the lines of "When we know better, we can (and should) do better." We are now able to image the brain and observe neural excitation patterns in real time through the technology of functional MRI (fMRI) and electrocorticography. Most of us have probably heard various theories that humans are not currently utilizing the full capacity of our brainpower, and we all might fantasize about unlocking this supposedly vast potential and the new skills we might acquire as a result. Personally, I would be happy with small improvements that could potentially make humans happier and more content in their daily lives. Having a better conception of how our brain manages through understanding our basic human instincts should help us find a better path toward positive behaviour modification.

When we are coaching high-performance athletes, we often try to have them clear their mind and relax before attempting a difficult movement or task. Game day or competition time is not the occasion to change techniques or teach something new. You will often see inexperienced coaches trying this during a panic situation, or when their team is losing badly. This strategy most often results in escalating frustration from the athletes and even worse execution of athletic skills, leaving everyone feeling terribly disappointed, and even more so when they lose the game.

We can find examples of this in business as well. Many of the business advisers we have worked with at Totum Life Science have always emphasized that when things get tough, do not let the actions of your competition guide your fundamental decisions. Do not panic and adjust everything as a reaction to your stress. Work hard, stay the course and do what you do best. When you think of brands that have withstood the test of time and are still successful, such as Microsoft, Apple, Nike or even the iconic fashion house Chanel, there is a common theme of consistent messaging and brand confidence.

This reliable pathway helps everyone feel comfortable in their environment because we know what to expect, and that understanding allows us to feel more relaxed and assured that we can have a certain level of trust in the outcome. In athletics, we often refer to this idea when we compare an older, experienced athlete with a younger, inexperienced one. When we have executed a skill in a stressful environment thousands of times, it can become part of our subconscious

Having a better conception of how our brain manages through understanding our basic human instincts should help us find a better path toward positive behaviour modification.

———————

pathway and we can be confident in our ability to do what we need to do without "overthinking" things. If we are new to a situation, our brain is taking in tons of external information as we try to determine the best way to accomplish what we need to do. The processing required as we attend to vast amounts of information slows down our reaction time significantly. It can even have an impact on our overall muscle tension, ultimately decreasing our ability to perform at our best.

I recall a time, in my early days of coaching, when I was trying to recruit a young sprinter to our track team. After many weeks and multiple conversations, I had convinced him to come and "just try" an indoor track practice. Two additional coaches who were extremely excited about his potential joined us. During high school, this talented athlete had been one of the fastest sprinters in our city. The draw of football and hockey was much stronger for him, so he stopped competing in track. After a couple of serious concussions in hockey, he had decided to leave that sport, and I was hoping he would consider sprinting again.

He had never used starting blocks for his races, so we wanted to see how he would make out with them, knowing that this could be a great way to enhance his overall speed in races. Plus, most sprinters find working on their "starts" a fun part of practice. We got him set up in the blocks and tried a few start sprints to 30 metres. Things looked quite good and you could feel the excitement growing amongst the coaches. Then we all started to give him feedback about things he should change or adjust. We did this to the point that on one start, his final one of the day, his brain was obviously trying very hard to process *way too much* information and he pushed out of the starting blocks into a complete face plant. The coaches were frozen and speechless for a moment as they tried to process what had just happened. We had never seen this before and we quickly rushed over to make sure this young athlete was okay. He did not suffer any external injuries, other than a bit of road rash to his chest. However, he was terribly embarrassed by what had happened, and you could tell as he looked around the track to see who else had witnessed this that the more serious damage was in his mind.

I glanced across to the other two coaches as we helped him up. We realized that we had basically coached someone right into a face plant by giving way too much technical advice at the same time. Completely stupid and ineffective. This young athlete eventually began laughing, much to our relief. We immediately realized that one coach speaking to him at a time would be more than enough to help him become a better sprinter.

We all have instinctive movement patterns that we are born with, and every good coach knows that your best pathway to success is to work within these pathways to enhance them. As exemplified by the story of our young track athlete, we should not try to change too many parts of the instinctive movement patterns at once, and rarely should we make these changes during a competitive situation. On game day we will always have greater success if we relax, clear our mind and let our subconscious movement patterns do what they were designed to do.

"Less is more" is often the best approach when teaching physical tasks, especially if you are trying to change a movement pattern that someone has been doing in an instinctual way for many years. The best coaches identify positive movement patterns in young athletes and then work with the inherent patterns to enhance and strengthen the athlete to an elite level. I believe this same analogy can be used for many of our instinctual behaviours. We should understand that they exist; and instead of fighting against them, our best and most efficient strategy is to enhance them and learn why they exist and how they are useful to us in our everyday life.

If we believe that our instinctive patterns and subconscious pathways are faster and sometimes "smarter" than our cognitive processes, it should be a goal to find ways to use them more, or even enhance them.

Instincts in Science

Part of what makes understanding our instincts so fascinating is that we do not have an exact, concrete definition of "instinct." Everyone perceives their instincts in a slightly different way. When we study animals both within and outside their natural habitats, we consistently find repeatable instinctual behaviours that have now been documented for hundreds of years.

Ivan Pavlov immediately comes to mind. Pavlov was a Nobel Prize–winning scientist who dedicated his life to research and has even described his intellectual curiosity as an "Instinct for Research." Many of his influential scientific breakthroughs were dependent on the consistent physiological responses of his dogs to varied external stimuli. By altering these stimuli and adapting unconscious responses in the dogs, he was able to modify various behaviours, leading to many psychological breakthroughs in the area now known as classical conditioning. In his lab, Pavlov was one of the first scientists able to demonstrate repeatable responses to external stimuli and then alter the stimuli in order to influence the responses. You could define some of these responses as "instinctual" because the animal responding was unaware of their behaviour; they also may be called "subconscious" responses and even, in some cases, simply "physiological" reactions. However we choose to label the response, the most important thing to understand is that our brains, and the brains of most living organisms, have defined pathways that lead to certain behaviours or actions. Some of these behaviours and actions are beneficial and some are not. When we understand these subconscious pathways better and when we learn how to either enhance or de-emphasize them, we will improve our ability to control our own outcomes and essentially harness the power that is already there.

Now that I may have completely confused you by combining a bunch of terms from behavioural science, let's go back to some basic definitions of "instinct."

Definition from a psychological viewpoint:

INSTINCT—Is the inherent disposition of a living organism toward a particular behaviour.

Instincts are generally inherited.

Instinctive behaviour can be demonstrated across much of the broad spectrum of animal life.

One of my favourite definitions comes from the *Merriam-Webster* dictionary:

[Instinct is] a largely inheritable and unalterable tendency of an organism to make a complex and specific response to environmental stimuli without involving reason.

Researcher Mark S. Blumberg published a comprehensive article explaining how our ideas or understanding of instinct has more recently evolved.

How do migratory birds, herding dogs, and navigating sea turtles do the amazing things that they do? For hundreds of years, scientists and philosophers have struggled over possible explanations. In time, one word came to dominate the discussion: *instinct*. It became the catch-all explanation for those adaptive and complex abilities that do not obviously result from learning or experience. Today, various animals are said to possess a survival instinct, migratory instinct, herding instinct, maternal instinct, or language instinct. But a closer look reveals that these and other "instincts" are not satisfactorily described as inborn, pre-programmed, hardwired, or genetically determined. Rather, research in this area teaches us that species-typical behaviors *develop*—and they do so in

Our brains, and the brains
of most living organisms,
have defined pathways
that lead to certain
behaviours or actions.

————————

every individual under the guidance of species-typical experiences occurring within reliable ecological contexts.

Blumberg goes on to explain why many of these definitions can cause confusion within the structure of science and research:

The more we dive into these matters, the harder it is to settle on any clear notion of what an instinct actually is. As Patrick Bateson has pointed out, this conceptual confusion about instinct is reflected in the many meanings that are routinely ascribed to it, including:

- Present at birth
- Not learned
- Developed before it is used
- Unchanged once developed
- Shared by all members of a species
- Adapted during evolution
- Served by a distinct module in the brain
- Attributable to genes

… No one doubts the existence of species-typical behaviors, and we can all agree that any science of behavior must endeavor to make sense of them. But there is an unsettling gulf between widely accepted assumptions surrounding instinct and the actual science available to explain it.

Lack of a clear definition can lead to confusion when we try to understand how our instincts influence our behaviours. When we add to this the influences related to different cultures, belief systems and sometimes even religions, the discrepancies make understanding the science more difficult.

Terms Used Interchangeably with "Instinct"

While researching this book, I uncovered many terms used throughout science, literature and even current media that refer to behaviours that are interchangeable with "instinct."

- Human nature
- Innate drives
- Ancient drives
- Human reactions
- Innate actions
- Genetically determined behaviours
- Human desires
- Subconscious actions
- Intuition
- Human drives
- Inherent actions
- Natural reflexes

To confuse matters even more, Blumberg goes on to explain that the current evidence points to an increased likelihood that "our natures are acquired," speculating that we do not yet have a full understanding of human and animal behaviours as they relate to our instincts and that our previous definitions are probably too simplistic. In other words, "nurture" has a larger influence than "nature."

The part of Blumberg's research that I find most exciting is the idea that we probably have vast potential to improve and alter our basic instinctual patterns, and ultimately advance our behaviours in many ways to improve our life. We have endless examples of this when we look at the behaviours of high-performers throughout history, and our future generations will continue to surpass these levels as they always have. It is important to understand why these enhancements occur from a neurological and physiological level, but because many of our behaviours are linked to our psychology, we cannot ignore this important variable.

Based on these definitions, it seems that our instincts probably have a direct link to our subconscious thought processes. The main difference I see is that our instincts will often have a direct effect on driving our behaviour, whereas our subconscious thoughts may or may not result in specific actions or feelings. I agree with Blumberg that our instincts are adaptable, and I also agree with Gladwell that once we have a better understanding of how our brain functions, it is our responsibility to act on these learnings.

TRAINING TOOL: Improving Our Instinctual Behaviours by Understanding Them Better

By understanding that our instincts are complex patterns of behaviour we are born with, and that these patterns are susceptible to change through the influence of our environment and experiences, we can refine them to the best of our ability. We do not want to push against our instinctual patterns or actions; instead, we should learn to enhance them to our personal advantage, using them as a launching point for our further development or performance. For example, walking and running are instinctual movement patterns that we are born with. Once we learn how to do these things adequately, we usually stop trying to learn about them and are satisfied with "good enough." What if we spent a bit of extra time, maybe working with a professional coach, looking at our gait analysis, to try to improve our techniques for both skills? Chances are the results of this extra effort would be well worth it over a lifetime. Similarly, there are many times as children when we try to run as fast as we possibly can. This is an excellent way to train our bodies and our brains to become more efficient at this instinctual movement pattern. Once we reach a certain age, though, we stop trying to run as fast as possible, and consequently our ability or "instinct" to run fast is greatly diminished—a perfect example of the "use it or lose it" phenomenon. For most of us, there is no specific day or time or age when we decide not to run fast anymore; it just gradually creeps up on us as our lives become more busy with sedentary demands or options. Instead, we should make a point of regularly trying to run as fast as possible, no matter what age we are. It is great for our overall health and a good way to prevent early decline of our neuromuscular systems.

Another good example would be working on our instinctual ability to communicate. We all learn to communicate effectively when we are young. This learning is initially motivated by our survival instinct, so we can tell our parents or caregivers what we want and need. As we get older, we improve our ability to communicate so we can talk with our teachers, partners, friends and possibly bosses or co-workers. Then most of us will reach a plateau in this skill. However, we know there are many people who continue to grow in this area. They may become world-famous leaders as their speeches resonate and inspire populations for years to come; they may be hired at a prestigious university because their lectures motivate the next generation of thinkers; or a great communicator could find themselves famous almost overnight through podcasts and YouTube. If we accept that our instinctual patterns have the ability to be enhanced, we will open up a whole new level of possibilities for our personal performance.

RECOMMENDED READING: *Blink: The Power of Thinking without Thinking* by Malcolm Gladwell

4

Working with vs. Working against Our Instincts

The prairie was forever, with its wind whispering through the long, dead grasses, through the long and endless silence. Winter came and spring and fall, then summer and winter again; the sun rose and set again, and everything that was once—was again—forever and forever.

W.O. MITCHELL,
WHO HAS SEEN THE WIND

I WAS BORN IN 1968 in a hospital in Saskatoon. My family on both sides were farmers going back a couple of generations. As a child growing up on a prairie farm, my main goal was to get outside to play, every day, for as many hours as humanly possible. Inside meant that you would be asked to help out around the house and join in meal preparation. Outside meant freedom. Once I understood this rhythm, I masterminded my escape every single day... even in the rain and snow.

My usual summer routine on our prairie farm included waking up mid-morning and slowly making my way into the kitchen, usually to find it completely empty as my feet padded across the cool floors of a quiet farmhouse. My mom would already be outside working in the garden and my dad would have left for his work in the fields many hours earlier. My brother and I were basically left to fend for ourselves during the day. We would make ourselves breakfast and eventually wander outside to explore what was happening in the farmyard. Normally, we didn't want our parents to catch sight of us, because that meant we would be given some type of outside chore, such as gardening, pulling weeds or mowing the lawn.

There were a few special days every year when things happened a bit differently. Occasionally, as the prairie sunlight was just starting to rise through the windows, my dad would come into my room and whisper, "Time to go..." I knew that I needed to quickly get some clothes together and come to the kitchen. I would sit at the kitchen counter and eat the small breakfast he had prepared for me. He would have had his breakfast a while ago, often around 4:30 a.m., as he waited for a reasonable time to wake me up. To him, "reasonable" would be between 5:30 and 6 a.m. While I ate, he would prepare our lunch for the day; our favourite was sandwiches made with home-made bread slathered with Cheez Whiz, sliced onions and tons of salt and pepper. A couple of bottles of Coke and some chocolate bars would always be hidden under the down-filled coats in the truck. They were stored there to prevent them from melting in the hot mid-day sun, and to my surprise this technique always worked. By the time we piled into his Chevy half-ton, the sky was a blindingly bright blue and the green ground was still covered with dew. We would pull out of the yard slowly, tires crunching on the gravel. I would have remained still and silent this whole time, hoping not to wake anyone else in the family. I cherished our alone time, and I did not want my younger brother to suddenly wake up and ask to tag along.

We always had to take a long route to get where we were going. My dad would pull over and roll down his window to look at our crops. He would explain something about them to me, but I often was not really listening. I disliked this part of the drive because I found it boring compared to where we were headed. I felt as though I had looked at these fields a million times, and each year it was basically the same old wheat field. Dad would explain to me, often at length, what was happening in the crops at certain points of interest. I would nod my head in apparent understanding, hoping he would put his foot down on the accelerator and we would be back to flying over the dirt roads, leaving our dust trail behind.

Finally, we would turn north, and I would sit up in my seat, scan-ning the horizon for any form of animal life, any slight movement across the vast open fields. Antelope were common, white-tailed deer not as much. If I was able to spot them before Dad did, that was a great moment. He did not miss much, but he would be impressed with my ability to find the animals, often repeating with amazement, "I do not know how you saw that!"

As we continued to drive north, the flat prairie changed into beautiful green rolling hills. The community simply referred to this area as "The River Hills." These velvety slopes surrounded the South Saskatchewan River on both sides and formed coulees in the middle of flatlands and farmers' fields. All species of animals loved the coulees because of their shelter, abundant food and access to water. Dad, being an expert hunter, knew where to find them all. We would spend almost a full day in the coulees, hiking the thin dirt trails that were made by deer and cattle. Dad would quietly narrate our findings and what they meant. He would pick berries and sage and mash them up in his hand, then give them to me as their strong cedar smell filled the air. We would flush out partridges, hawks and sometimes pheasants. Dad would warn me as we approached a bush that the birds were there, but I always felt as though I was going to have a heart attack when they suddenly flew out, wings beating so close beside us we could practically feel them. Those were the best days with my dad, and I cherished that time in nature with him.

These hikes with my dad could only take place when there was a rare break in the farming work that needed to be done. In the spring, before planting, we loved watching the water run off the hills into the riverbed. In the middle of summer, during the main growing period, there would be a couple of days off where we could continue our hiking adventure. Then there might be some brief moments in the fall if harvest was done early, but this all ended during hunting season.

The southwest corner of Saskatchewan has always been a prime location for duck and goose hunting. Avid hunters from all over North America would descend on our farm every fall, parking their expensive RVs all over the property. Dad would take them to various places surrounding our properties to hunt geese, ducks, partridges, deer and even the occasional moose.

I hated hunting season.

As a child growing up on a prairie farm, my main goal was to get outside to play, every day, for as many hours as humanly possible.

———————

I felt a strong sense of betrayal from my dad during this season, as I rooted for the animals I had fallen in love with during the spring and summer months. The animals we had admired during our hiking adventures were now at risk of being killed for sport and food, with my dad leading the way. Since he was a Junior Canadian Trap Shooting Champion, I was confident that any animal within his range would not survive. As the hunters returned home with their kill from each day, I could tell by their joyful chatter that they had all made their quotas for the season. Sometimes I would even suggest to them that if they had made their quota already, they should probably just pack up and leave. They rarely heeded my suggestion.

Hunting season in our community would last for approximately a month. Although it was a very social time, with many newcomers visiting our small town, I basically scowled at my dad any chance I got. I also may have mentioned to a few of the hunters that when I inherited this farmland from my dad, I was going to turn it all into a bird sanctuary!

Unfortunately, that never happened.

The Breakdown

When I was in grade five, my mom let us know that she was going back to teaching full-time. This meant that we would live in Saskatoon during the school year and live on the farm only during the summer holidays. I enjoyed my life in the city, but my emotional attachment to the farm was much greater. I spent a few days crying and protesting and then, as children usually do, I adapted to the change.

I not only adapted—I soon began to thrive in the city. I joined every sports team that would have me. My marks improved significantly because I was not changing schools twice a year, and based on the standardized testing scores I was invited to be part of a program at our school for academically talented students. My peers at school became my close friends, and soon I did everything humanly possible to avoid leaving my exciting life in the city for the "boring" farm. I purposely ignored everything I had learned about nature because it reminded me of the farm, and instead I immersed myself in training for various sports.

When I turned 16, I convinced my parents that I had to stay in the city and train all summer, but they decided that in order to do that, I would have to get a job. I applied for many jobs and settled on three that would occupy all my time outside training, just to ensure I did not have to go back to the farm.

I continued with these obsessive, determined behaviours through high school and even into my first degree at university. I had decided that city life was the only life for me. Keep in mind that Saskatoon has a population of around 200,000, so it is not exactly a major metropolis, but it is massive compared with a farm located outside a town of a couple of hundred locals. Other than noticing the occasional sunset on a particularly stunning Saskatchewan night, I basically ignored all signs of nature on purpose. Years would go by between hikes with my dad, and I would explain to him that I had other priorities to attend to. Farming and hiking were not a part of my overall plan and would not help me reach any of my new life goals.

Looking back, I can say that my health suffered greatly during that time. I was constantly training, so I was getting more than enough exercise, but my nutrition consisted of tons of processed foods. Pasta with a jar of tomato sauce was my go-to meal. My weight fluctuated regularly, and I was always tired and using caffeine, even in pill form, to try to stay awake and accomplish everything that needed to be done during a typical day. I seemed to go from one injury to another, and had to visit the University Athletic Therapy Room regularly—so often, in fact, that I was given my own key and taught how to use the ultrasound machine myself, so I could do my own therapy after the clinic was closed. Many times each year, my body would simply "shut down." I would usually be diagnosed with a strep infection and be forced to take a couple of days off. I would walk over to the student health centre, get my usual course of antibiotics and rush right back into my hectic routine.

They say that when you know better, you do better. As I look back on those crazy years, I am filled with sadness as I wonder about what could have been. During so many of those important training years, I did not know what I do now about health, nutrition and self-care. Had I known that my immune system would have benefited greatly from even just a small amount of proper rest, better nutrition and some time spent relaxing in nature, my path as an athlete would have been drastically enhanced.

My life continued in this extreme way for at least a decade. At one point I had a full class schedule and approximately five part-time jobs. I was training with the university swim team in the morning (because of persistent injuries, they would not allow me to run), and then I was heading to track practice in the late afternoon to try to work on my throwing events and whatever else I could do without aggravating my current injuries.

I basically forced myself into a level of discipline where I was able to ignore most of my basic instincts. I was chronically lacking sleep, my stress levels were extreme and constant, my nutrition was mostly deficient, and I was basically functioning on pure adrenalin and caffeine to keep up with the demands of my busy schedule. At the same time, I was a highly motivated person and was driven by a system that rewarded high marks and a strong work ethic.

My athletic career ended too quickly, owing to injuries.

One of my most focused goals was to compete in the Canada Games, representing Saskatchewan as a heptathlete, the year it was being hosted in Saskatoon. I even decided to take the year off from competing for the university team so that I could focus on my rehabilitation along with additional intense training all through the winter season. As soon as spring came and I got back into speed training and actual competing, my injuries returned.

Instead of participating in the Canada Games that summer, I watched my teammates and close friends compete as I sat in the stands wearing a half-leg cast. I was still working on campus as a research assistant. Every day I would see athletes from all over the country leaving the athletes' village residences, heading off to their various practices or events. It was devastating for me because I would be graduating soon and this would have been one of my final competitive athletic events. Instead of taking part as an athlete, I was simply a spectator.

Most of my teammates had amazing performances that year, because we had all been involved in extra training programs to help us get ready to represent the host city. I was truly happy for everyone, and thrilled at how well Saskatchewan was doing at these games, but for every day of the track events I had to drag myself there, with crutches and cast, to cheer everyone on. Eventually it got too difficult and I stopped going. I avoided the closing ceremonies and did my best to ignore all the talk about the parties that followed. It was the opposite of the outcome I had worked incredibly hard for. Once the cast was removed, I was very committed (again) to getting back to rehab, and I even tried one more season at the track, but nothing was ever the same. My ankle was still in pain every day and I knew it was time to stop the constant aggravation.

Often the best lessons in life come when things do not go as we had planned, or when we are not actually seeing the results we hoped for, and instead of reaching our goals, we are faced with failure. I am very familiar with failure, and although it would take many years for me to understand what I was doing wrong during those years, this information has become an important part of my success and has contributed to the accomplishments of the athletes, clients and patients I work with today.

When it comes to our health, our performance and our happiness, so many times the answers we are looking for are inside us. We just need to take the time to figure them out.

When it comes to our
health, our performance
and our happiness, so many
times the answers we are
looking for are inside us.

———————

Creating the Right Environment

The way we structure our environment has a huge impact on our overall health and performance. Even the simple things in our lives, such as what time we go to bed, when we wake up, our exercise schedule, and our strategy for stress relief are part of our environment. I evaluate all these components in more detail in later chapters, but it is essential to your success to take a step back and analyze the environment you have created for your life. In the stories I have recounted, it is eminently clear that my health (both mental and physical) thrived during the years I was living on our farm. I was rarely sick, I enjoyed eating nutritious food often picked straight from our garden, I competed in various sports and I was never injured. As my life moved to the city, and I ignored nature, I made poor choices related to nutrition and I was constantly sleep deprived. My health suffered greatly. I realize that it is not practical to say that you must live in a rural environment to have good health and perform better, but I use my story as an example of two opposite ways of living. There are many ways to incorporate a structure or environment in which to exist that will enhance your instincts instead of ignoring them.

TRAINING TOOL: Work with Your Instincts

It is helpful to look for both good and bad patterns in your life. If you can reflect on days when you had lots of energy and felt extra-productive, try to notice what was common to those days. In comparison, on days when everything went completely backwards and fell apart, can you find similarities in the events leading up to those days? There is a good chance that on your best days, you were doing things that aligned with your instinctual habits and needs, such as getting a good night's rest, or spending more time outside and less time on devices.

Similarly, if you are noticing regular "breakdowns" in your health, it is worth further analysis to see if there is anything you can change to prevent these negative outcomes. If you find that you get sick constantly, you are probably suffering from a diminished immune system. Work together with your health care providers to figure out what you need to change to improve your personal situation. These details are for you to discover. A journal can help tremendously with this process. Look for patterns and then try to repeat the good days and find a better understanding of what things in your external environment make you feel better and perform well.

RECOMMENDED READING: *Who Has Seen the Wind* by W.O. Mitchell

5

Modern Life and Its Impact on Our Instincts

Trust your instinct to the end,
though you can render no reason.

RALPH WALDO EMERSON

T HE FIRST MCDONALD'S franchise opened on April 15, 1955. Suddenly, food became fast and required no effort for us to prepare it, serve it or clean up after we were finished. Forget about hunting and foraging—life for human beings had changed forever.

Today, in many larger centres, we can have almost any type of food or alcohol delivered to our doorstep within minutes, along with any other items of daily living we might want or need. Most of our daily communication is done via computer or cellphone, and in some cases we are connected to these devices for over 12 hours a day. Our main forms of entertainment are also brought right into our homes, often through these same devices. Most work environments require more or less constant use of a computer or cellphone, and most humans now spend way too many hours sitting, or at least with limited movement, while at work.

How are these drastic lifestyle changes affecting us on a physical level? We have done very well over the last couple of hundred years, but we are currently hitting a ceiling when it comes to the health of our populations and our overall life expectancy. In the United States we have seen reports that life expectancy has decreased for the past three years in a row. As our world has dealt with the COVID-19 pandemic, we have also come to understand that many of the deaths associated with the virus were related to comorbidities brought on by lifestyle choices, such as smoking, obesity, diabetes and cardiovascular disease. The increase in deaths from what have been labelled the "diseases of despair"—drug overdose, suicide and alcoholism—along with lower respiratory illnesses, deaths from the flu, Alzheimer's, diabetes and stroke are presented as possible explanations for the overall decreases in life expectancy.

In North America we are still seeing a rise in obesity along with the diseases associated with metabolic disorders. Scientists and doctors are now able to keep people with heart disease, stroke and diabetes alive longer thanks to rapidly developing surgical techniques and drug protocols. At the same time, we are seeing dramatic increases in the incidence of depression and mental health issues, especially when we look at younger age groups. There have also been surveys designed to evaluate the new gig economy, specifically looking at "quality of life" measures. These large-scale studies indicate that loneliness is a common problem across all age groups in North America. It is obvious why we should be worried about these findings. We know that loneliness has a major influence on our overall health, but more than that, it significantly impacts our happiness and quality of life.

In our rapidly changing world, we now have technology that will easily perform many jobs better than humans. We have 3-D printers that can actually print food or guns, along with virtual reality systems that can transport us to basically anywhere we would like to be. Humans should be thriving, ecstatic and "living our best lives," but the research shows otherwise. What are we missing?

A Very Personal Case Study

My dad had become quite ill from a few major health problems. To help you understand these issues better, I will go back a few years. In 2001, I had a call from my mom letting me know that she and my dad were going to divorce. Although this news was devastating to me, it did not come as a complete surprise. They were leading very separate lives, with my dad living mainly on the farm and my mom working full-time in the city. Their split was amicable but meant that parts of the farm would need to be divided and sold. My dad was an excellent farmer and a terrible accountant. In retrospect, I am sure that with his grade ten education he often had no idea what was happening with his farm in a financial sense. There were many examples of this through the years, with grand ideas and expensive equipment purchases that eventually led to him declaring bankruptcy a few years after the divorce. With his farmland gone, he still needed an income, and so he decided that the best option was to drive a grain truck and work for other farming operations he knew in the community.

You may be wondering, what does this story have to do with instinct? Just bear with me.

My dad's lifestyle changed dramatically. He was now spending long hours sitting in his truck, often driving through stressful weather conditions, always on a strict timeline, trying to get as many loads finished in a day as possible. He would grab food on the go, eating at the closest fast-food place in whatever town he was passing through. Because he was now single and living by himself on the farm, his daily needs were basic and no one was monitoring how he was eating, sleeping or exercising.

His health deteriorated gradually, as it normally does with these types of lifestyle changes. I would check with him about his eating and exercise, but my advice (possibly preaching) only went so far. The first sign of more serious problems was that his sleeping became extremely limited and erratic. This went on for a few years, and then one night my phone rang at 3 a.m. and the voice on the other end was an ER doctor telling me that my dad was being airlifted to the emergency department of the Saskatoon Royal University Hospital. He'd had a heart attack.

He was rushed into surgery as I rushed to the Toronto airport to get on the next plane to Saskatoon. I arrived at the hospital the next day. I

In nature, when we
encounter a stressful
situation, our first
instinct is to move, usually
as fast as possible,
away from the danger.

———————

will never forget what one of the very experienced nurses said to me about his case. She looked up from her chair and said, "You have no idea how many truck drivers we get in here with serious heart problems."

My dad made a speedy recovery from his heart surgery and was back at his busy work schedule within weeks. As I flew back to Toronto, trying to think of some solutions to help my dad, this statement from the nurse weighed heavily on me. I am positive that the reason they see so many truck drivers suffering from heart disease is that the career and way of life of a truck driver are structured exactly opposite to how we should be functioning as human beings. Our bodies were never designed to be sitting, basically immobilized for many hours of the day, while we encounter stressful situations through our visual, auditory and kinesthetic systems. In nature, when we encounter a stressful situation, our first instinct is to move, usually as fast as possible, away from the danger. The job of driving a truck means that you will spend your day encountering various stresses, and yet you will remain seated during all of them. This is the opposite of an environment designed to enhance your instincts. Another way to think about this could be an image of a wild animal, such as a coyote. What if we taught coyotes to drive motorcycles? They could use this method for their hunting. The initial concept might be interesting, because they would be much faster at hunting and each catch would take less of their own energy. As with humans and our vehicles, what if you then told them they could *only* be on the motorcycle and they had to use it for *all* of their daily activities? We would probably be left with some very out-of-shape, unhealthy coyotes!

There is a famous study by Jeremy Morris, published in the *Lancet* in 1953, of London double-decker bus employees, comparing the health of the drivers, who sat all day, with the conductors or ticket takers, who were basically standing and walking for most of the day. As you would suspect, the bus drivers' health suffered greatly because of their sedentary lifestyle and often stressful job. They had much higher rates of cardiovascular disease, along with cancer, and lower life expectancy. When they were compared with the ticket takers, the drivers' incidence of chronic disease was significantly higher even though, outside their work environments, both test groups led very similar lifestyles.

I have read many media headlines claiming that "sitting is the new smoking" and I believe this to be devastatingly true. It was certainly the case for our family. When my dad went back to work after his heart attack, he did improve some of his lifestyle habits for a while, with better eating and more regular exercising. His sleeping patterns were still a problem because of stress and long work hours, but he was walking more regularly and some days he would even jog around the dirt roads surrounding his small farm. But my dad's new pattern of health problems, followed by emergency trips to Saskatoon by either myself or my brother, would repeat itself many times.

A few years after my dad's heart attack, on a typical weekday, one of our admin team at Totum came out to the gym floor to tell me there was a person on the phone for me, calling from my dad's farm. This had never happened before, so I rushed to the phone to hear one of our dear friends tell me that he had found my dad sitting in his truck in the ditch, completely disoriented.

Dad's heart surgery had been followed closely by a diagnosis of stomach cancer and another surgery, and then chemotherapy and radiation treatments. Feeling a constant pressure and need to return to work, he continued to push himself to the absolute limit in order to carry out his daily tasks. My dad at this time was in his mid-70s and somehow, through stubborn determination, he still managed to show up and work and usually make it through each day with a high level of accomplishment. Some days, though, he did not make it through and ended up in the ditch, disoriented. I attribute his ability to push himself for so long to the fact that, prior to driving a truck, he had enjoyed decades of a very healthy lifestyle, including an active work-day with farming, many active leisure activities, healthy eating, and strong connections to his family and community.

When we ignore our basic survival instincts, including our instinct to live in a way that our body was designed for, we may be okay for a while, but eventually our mental and physical health will deteriorate and we will regret that we ignored the signals our body was sending us. In my dad's case, the first sign was the disrupted sleeping. The second big sign was his heart attack, and the third significant sign was his abdominal cancer.

Having survived two major health events, Dad was still pushing through his exhausting work demands and not sleeping enough. Financial stress coupled with poor daily health habits continued to be a part of his regular routine. I was aware that this stress was having a detrimental impact on his relationships with his friends and his community. Regular phone conversations with me and my brother dissolved into arguments. We were often asked to lend him money for various overdue bills and sometimes even groceries. Alienating yourself from your closest relationships is another behaviour that goes against your basic instincts, and it also has a terribly negative impact on your overall health.

As Dad's health continued its downward spiral, I decided I would have to physically intervene. I called a couple of his doctors and scheduled examinations with his cardiologist for his heart and with his oncologist to ensure he was still cancer free. Dad's usual habit was to drive from his farm to his doctors' appointments (approximately 475 kilometres/300 miles) and then drive back home that night so he could be at work the next day. I knew that the only way I could convince him to stay overnight and rest was to be there with him. By this point he was feeling too tired to argue with me. So I again found myself booking a flight back to Saskatoon.

We had a good visit the first day I was there. We ate at some of our favourite restaurants and walked around Saskatoon. As we strolled through the city that day, he tired much more easily than normal, and he mentioned a couple of times that his feet felt very heavy. We had dinner close to the hotel, and I begged him to eat as much as possible because he had recently lost so much weight, but he just did not have any appetite. We walked slowly back to the hotel, and as he was getting ready for bed, I watched him carefully and painfully take off his shoes and socks with so much effort and lots of heavy sighs. I was horrified when I saw his feet. I am not a general practitioner, nor do I know much about cardiology from a diagnostic perspective, but I had spent many years working in cardiac rehab as part of the exercise team. I was convinced that his massively swollen feet and black-and-blue toenails were indicative of bad news related to his heart, likely congestive heart failure. In all of the doctors' appointments he had been to over the past month, at no point had anyone given him a full physical exam to try to determine why he was feeling so poorly. The treatment plans were always about adjusting and usually adding medications, or basically just telling him that his symptoms were part of getting old and that he should slow down and not work so much.

I knew that rest would be the best thing for my dad at this point. He fell asleep immediately, but his loud breathing, coughing and choking kept me awake the whole night. I made some calls to try to find a cardiologist who would see him on short notice, but nobody was available, so when he eventually woke up, I got him into his big farm truck and off we went to the closest emergency ward.

Our wait at the Royal University Hospital that day was over eight hours. Dad was exhausted by the whole experience and the stress of waiting, and I was exhausted from the constant negotiating, worrying, and having to repeat his medical history over and over again all day long. That night, he was finally admitted to the cardiology ward. I felt he would be fine until the morning, so I left the hospital and drove back to the hotel. I collapsed into bed and awoke to the bright prairie sunlight streaming into the room. I felt as though I must have overslept, but of course it was only about 7 a.m. I went back to the hospital and met with the cardiology team, who explained that my dad was experiencing symptoms of congestive heart failure but that the diuretics had worked well last night and he was now able to move around with much less fluid in his lower extremities.

As usual, my dad was in great spirits. He loved talking to anyone who would listen about farming and his many outdoor adventures. He was excited to tell me where the various nurses were from and what rural communities they had connections to. Because of his extensive hours spent on the road, he knew all about these places in quite impressive detail. I listened to him give yet another general history to the attending nurse, and as he explained that he worked full-time driving a grain truck, it almost broke my heart when he said he needed at least five more years of work to become financially stable and pay off his debts. The largest ones were to me and my brother, and we never expected repayment, but I knew that he wished he would someday be able to do that. At this time, Dad appeared to be a healthy 77-year-old, and based on what he told the nurse, he would need to work a full-time schedule driving a truck until he was 82 years old. I silently thought to myself, "Unless he completely changes his lifestyle, that will never happen."

My flight back to Toronto was scheduled for that afternoon. I met with the team that would be working with my dad and it seemed as though they had a good plan in place for his recovery. I called his friends at the farm and let everyone know what was happening. It was a sad goodbye for me, but I was sure he would be feeling much better soon. I made him promise that he would eat as much as possible and leave the hospital bed to walk many times a day. He vowed to stick to that program.

I flew back to Toronto and was so ecstatic to finally see my family that I basically burst into tears the minute I walked in the door. My kids loved their grandfather and the farm. They were all genuinely concerned about him. I did my best to calm everyone down and I let them know that their grandfather was doing his best to get better and get out of the hospital as fast as humanly possible. All of this was true, but deep down I was very worried.

I finally had a good night of rest, but the next morning would bring another extremely stress-filled day. I desperately needed to get outside for a walk; I felt that a "nature break" would clear my head and help me de-stress. I was hopeful that I could come up with a plan to help Dad and keep everything moving smoothly at home.

At this same time, my youngest son was suffering from debilitating bouts of anxiety. There were a couple of issues that could be linked to this development. I knew that my recent trips to Saskatchewan and the condition of his grandfather were not helpful. He had also just found out from a classmate at school that he had not made a Greater Toronto Hockey League (GTHL) team, which was by far the most important thing in his world. Because he received this bad news at school, he had now decided that going to school made him feel sick and he could no longer manage it. He missed so many days of school during this time, and we even had situations where we had to physically carry him to the school, where his amazing and understanding teacher would meet us outside and try to convince him to go in. Each time I was away in Saskatchewan helping my dad, his anxiety would get a bit worse.

When I woke up the morning after my return from Saskatoon, he immediately started complaining of an aching stomach. Any parent who has dealt with anxiety issues with their children will know this is always a bad sign; the days that start with stomach problems rarely end the way you would like them to. I tried to manage my son's complaints by staying positive and telling him he would soon feel better. He refused to eat breakfast. I literally had to drag him out the door, but I was hoping that a walk in the fresh air would change his feelings. However, his school was not that far away. Added to this was the fact that every few steps he would stop and refuse to take another step. I grew frustrated to the point where I told him his choice was school or the SickKids hospital. It was not my best parenting moment, possibly one of the worst. I also explained to him that I was incredibly sad and worried about his grandfather, so I just did not have it in me to argue

When we ignore our
basic survival instincts,
we may be okay for a
while, but eventually our
mental and physical
health will deteriorate.

———————

anymore. We were standing outside the school, he was crying, I was crying, and I decided to give up. We slowly walked home. The concept of the sandwich generation is a real thing, and I felt it deeply that day. I dropped my son off at home, bundled myself up, and grabbed the dog and went out for a long walk, feeling as though I had failed as a daughter because I had left my dad alone at the hospital in Saskatoon and that I was also failing as a parent.

After approximately one week, my dad talked his way out of the emergency department in Saskatoon and happily made his way back to the farm and back to work. He sounded great, and I knew he was thrilled to be back in his community and enjoying his time with the farming family he worked for.

Seven days later, I received a call saying he had been transferred by ambulance to the emergency department of a hospital in Medicine Hat. Dad's condition deteriorated extremely quickly. Within approximately four days he was in organ failure, and soon a decision was made to transfer him back to Saskatchewan for palliative care at his local hospital. Back at the Toronto airport, I caught the first flight I could get on and made my way to the small town of Leader, Saskatchewan. By the time I got to the hospital in Leader, my dad was barely able to talk, but we did communicate a bit. The hospital in Leader was quite different from our experience in Saskatoon. The staff all knew my dad; many of them had known him since they were young. They treated me like family and always welcomed his many visitors the same way. I was so appreciative of their care and how they treated both of us with amazing respect and kindness. I will never forget how good they were.

Within three days, he was gone.

I spent large parts of the days in Leader by myself, filled with regret and wondering what I could have done better for Dad. My final day there was spent in a quiet room at the small prairie hospital completely alone with my dad's lifeless body as I waited for the funeral home to come pick him up. The outpouring of grief and concern from his farming community was incredible, even overwhelming. I realized how lucky my dad was to have these deep and meaningful connections with these people. Everywhere I went in the town, from the pharmacy to my bed and breakfast to the local coffee shop, I was comforted and supported by people, many of whom I had just met during this visit.

For most of his life, my dad's lifestyle had many components that were immensely positive when we look at things from an instinctual level. Growing up in rural Saskatchewan, you could argue, offered an almost ideal way of life. He spent tons of time outdoors, was in constant motion for most of his day, was a great sleeper, and had wonderful relationships with his community and family. He enjoyed competing in activities such as baseball, golf and trap shooting, and even though he never went to church, he loved singing, so he volunteered for the church choir. Most of his diet growing up consisted of homemade food from a garden, or meat purchased directly from other farmers or ranchers. That lifestyle completely changed, however, when he was forced to sell his farm and started driving a grain truck full-time. The negative effects of his new unhealthy lifestyle did not take long to drastically alter his lifespan, along with his quality of life in his last decade.

After waiting for what seemed like forever at the hospital with my dad's body, I flopped back into my car and drove three and a half hours to Saskatoon, tears streaming down my face most of the way there. At the airport, I begged my way onto one of the only flights that would land in Toronto that night, at 3 a.m., in the middle of an ice storm.

The next three months at home were dismal. The weather in Toronto in late winter can suck the life out of anyone—weeks of grey days, blowing snow, moments of sunshine to get your hopes up, followed by more snow. On a more positive note, my youngest son now knew I was home for good and started to feel better. He was also seeing a fantastic counsellor and we were all learning better coping methods to help him manage his anxiety. The reality is that young people are now suffering from significantly higher levels of mental health issues compared with previous generations. You might argue that conditions such as anxiety, depression and ADHD have always been present in our young populations and that we are now just beginning to recognize and diagnose these problems, but the research suggests otherwise. According to the National Institute of Mental Health, nearly one in three adolescents aged 13 to 18 will experience an anxiety disorder. The National Survey of Children's Health reports that these numbers have been rising steadily; between 2007 and 2012, anxiety disorders in children and teens went up 20 percent.

The research on this topic carried out in the last two decades demonstrates a trend similar to the increases in mental health disease seen in adults, suggesting that many of these problems can be directly attributed to the hectic, over-programmed, overworked demands of our current lifestyle.

Our society has "evolved" in a way that is not as healthy for our younger generations as it could be. While we can all agree that organized sports are great for kids, the research overwhelmingly supports the concept of free play along with a multi-sport approach for younger ages. In a city the size of Toronto, I find that most of our young elite athletes are forced to "specialize" too soon. You can find parents and coaches who believe that if two practices a week are good, five will obviously be better. My youngest son and his reaction to the politics of the GTHL is a good example of this. In so many instances, organized sport for young athletes has been pushed forward in an extreme way that does not focus on the overall health of its younger participants. Parents with limited knowledge of best practices when it comes to long-term athlete development and the importance of a multi-sport approach for young children often feel pressured to add more training time (not to mention that most of these youth training enterprises are private and profit-driven). The parents are then left to deal with the negative repercussions that are the most common result.

TRAINING TOOL: Honouring Your Instincts in These Rapidly Evolving Times

You can ignore your instincts and live in a way that is detrimental to your health for a while. You may even find that by pushing yourself to maximum capacity every day, you will be a high achiever at your job or school or whatever external goals you are trying to accomplish. Eventually, though, something will break down. It will usually be related to your physical health, but sometimes the symptoms show up as mental health issues. The breakdowns may seem minor to start with, such as getting sick more easily, or finding that you are relying more on caffeine or other stimulants to get through your day—and then possibly alcohol, recreational drugs or sleeping pills to help you calm down and get to sleep at the end of the day. Problems with your regular sleep cycles are also a good indication that things are out of balance. If you ignore these initial signals and keep pushing forward, they will worsen, and the eventual results can be devastating.

These early, quieter signals are your body's way of telling you that something in the structure of your life needs to change. We have created lifestyles full of escapes and distractions that help us ignore these early signals: drugs or medications that mask our symptoms of discomfort, compelling Netflix series to fill our spare time, alcohol or stress eating to help us relax and various types of stimulants to help us keep going when we are exhausted. I have made great use of all of these several times over the course of my life, so I list them here completely without judgment. Science and epidemiological research on human health and longevity also demonstrate a clear path where these habits can devolve into much more serious problems. It is important to try to make even small positive changes before these habits grow into something more serious.

If you are having trouble pinpointing the exact problem or the cause of your feelings, this is a great time to seek the help of a professional counsellor. I have done this at many different stages in my life, and I am always amazed at how effective it can be. Often, even as I am explaining my current stressful situation to another trained professional, I can feel solutions forming in my brain. Regular check-ins with counsellors, mental health professionals and even life coaches can be extremely beneficial for both adults and children.

Children are not immune to the immense pressures that can arise from the values of our current North American lifestyle. I found the book *In Praise of Slow: Challenging the Cult of Speed* by Carl Honoré an inspirational and educational tool as a parent trying to manage in these often challenging environments, where we can feel constant pressure to accomplish so many things in a short period of time.

RECOMMENDED READING: *In Praise of Slow: Challenging the Cult of Speed* by Carl Honoré

6

Instincts to Survive—Human Evolution— Then and Now

That survival instinct, that will to live, that need to get back to life again, is more powerful than any consideration of taste, decency, politeness, manners, civility. Anything. It's such a powerful force.

DANNY BOYLE, DIRECTOR
OF *SLUMDOG MILLIONAIRE*

ONE OF THE main instincts that influences our health is our instinct for survival. This instinct motivates us to find food, shelter and water, and has a direct influence on many of our daily behaviours.

Some scientists believe that our survival instinct is also partially responsible for our preference or need to exist as members of a tribe, alongside other human beings. At some point in our evolution we would have realized that we were much stronger as part of a group. Our hunting and gathering abilities were vastly improved when we began doing these things with others. During this point in our history, we also were threatened by large animals. It is possible that in order to survive an encounter with these massive mammals, we needed a tribe of strong people to help us make it out alive, and hopefully end the encounter with some food to share with the group.

Yuval Noah Harari, in his recent book *Sapiens: A Brief History of Humankind*, cites our ability to connect, communicate and work together as a group as one of the main reasons *Homo sapiens* was able to defeat the much stronger and faster Neanderthals to become the dominant species on the planet. These instinctual behaviours probably have a much larger impact on our current health and survival than we have ever acknowledged, and sometimes we even do our best to ignore them in the hectic pace of our modern lifestyle.

Our survival instinct can drive us away from situations where we feel we might be injured or killed. There are very few people who would happily go walking outside in the middle of a hailstorm, or who would enjoy playing a round of golf as they witnessed lightning striking all around them. We have an instinct to build shelter or find shelter to protect us from our environment, and we also have difficulty falling asleep when we feel there might be danger close by. Humans are more tentative when we encounter darkness; you would probably have a hard time convincing anyone to enter an unknown, pitch-black forest in the middle of the night even if you could prove to them that there was no history of misadventure there.

On the surface, our high-tech, fast-paced modern lifestyle appears to bear little resemblance to the way our tribal ancestors lived. It is fascinating to realize that many of our behaviours related to our instincts for survival endure and have a powerful influence over our actions.

The level of motivation arising from our survival instincts can vary dramatically throughout our life. It is well documented that the brain of a teenage boy can sometimes be driven toward risky behaviours. At the same time, elderly people sometimes show up at their local hospital's emergency department because of dehydration. This is not usually owing to a shortage of drinking water, but is simply because their motivation to drink (and sometimes eat) has become greatly diminished, often with no apparent medical explanation.

Our instincts for survival also include a drive to rest and recover every day. However, the most recent research in sleep science indicates that in Western society we are a significantly under-slept population. We have evolved into a modern society with stimulants that are able to keep us awake much longer. Our busy schedules and constant accessibility through our array of electronic devices also fill many more hours of our day, thereby shrinking the hours we have available for proper rest and recovery.

To gain a better understanding of these instincts and how they work for us, it is best to start at the beginning. The earliest groups of

Homo sapiens were estimated to exist hundreds of thousands of years ago. These groups consisted mainly of foragers and hunters. Within these populations, people split into small groups or tribes to aid in the acquisition of food and for procreation. Their lives were lived in nature, and their survival was based on their ability to navigate a sometimes very hostile world. Tribes were formed to increase success rates when hunting for food and to better support each other in dangerous situations. Often these dangers came in the form of exceptionally large animals, and humans soon realized that if they worked together, they could defeat some of these creatures, while they would not survive if they remained alone.

The agricultural revolution began only 10,000 years ago. At that time, humans began to understand how to control plants and animal species, so they would have food available without having to hunt and forage daily for their nutritional requirements. Although the agricultural revolution led to a surplus of food in most cases, it also led to a life where schedules were controlled by the growing and harvesting requirements of agriculture. Instead of spending your days roaming through nature, you were now forced to stay in one area and tend to your crops.

Fast-forward several millennia. On October 14, 1878, Thomas Edison filed his first patent for the production of the electric light bulb, drastically augmenting our ability to be productive for many hours after darkness had fallen. Close to this same time, Alexander Graham Bell began developing the first telephone. This would allow us to communicate with other members of our community without leaving our homes. Communities were still thriving and working together to support each other, but we also clearly began to understand the concepts of "my property" or "my house." Families still lived together, but more commonly it was just a nuclear family within a single house or homestead. Socializing was important, and it was often done through religion or work, depending on where you had chosen to settle your family and build a home.

Our instincts for survival still have a large impact on how we exist every day.

———————

The first versions of the home refrigerator were invented around 1913. This meant that we did not need to immediately eat the animals we killed or the food we harvested; we could now store it for a while. Guns were used for many things at this time, including hunting. Agricultural advances had led to grocery stores filled with produce that we could now purchase at our convenience and store in our new refrigerator. Most of our communities or tribes would never have to forage and hunt for food again.

The Big Questions Related to Our Survival Instincts

When we are solving a problem scientifically, we should always start at the beginning and identify the variables we are interested in studying. We want to come up with a hypothesis that captures what we think should happen, along with alternate hypotheses that could explain other outcomes.

Our instincts for survival still have a large impact on how we exist every day. Our choices related to food, careers and where we live can all be sourced back to these basic instincts and the idea that we want to give ourselves the best chance for a long and prosperous life.

Here are some questions I believe will help us evaluate our current lifestyle choices on a more scientific basis, with the goal of improving our understanding of how our instincts affect our daily behaviours and ultimately our existence.

- Why do we act the way we do when our survival instincts identify fear?

- Why do our bodies seem to crave certain things even when they are not necessarily good for us?

- Why do we make certain choices about when we eat or what we eat?

- How do we decide whom to socialize with?

- Why are we a sleep-deprived society?

- Why are we not as physically active as we used to be?

- How do culture and ritual influence our health and well-being?

The following are questions we must ask ourselves regularly to understand our instincts:

- What happens if we ignore our instincts?

- How does this affect our mood and behaviours?

- Alternatively, if we understand that neural pathways related to our instincts exist in most humans, how can we enhance their development?

- In a time of massive technological development, how can we use our instincts to our advantage in everyday life?

These questions are important to answer if we are going to try to change our behaviours in order to live a healthier, more successful or even happier life. I believe that the answers to many of these questions are related to a rediscovery of our instincts, and that we are born with the neural pathways that cause various behaviours. For this reason, I also believe that if we understand these pathways and learn to work with them instead of against them, we will be healthier and perform better.

Instincts for Greed

There is a pathway or behavioural drive that is related to our survival instinct and can be best described as our instinct for greed or selfishness. In our current times, it can be a valuable instinct to try to understand and hopefully learn to control for the betterment of all humanity. There are many actions that we regularly observe, especially in today's political landscape, that can be attributed to our instinct for greed or selfishness.

I observe these behaviours regularly in my daily life: when I ask my children to help with things around the house, when I am interviewing for new positions on our team at Totum, and in many of my interactions with patients and clients during the day. The concept of "What's in it for me?" is a relevant identifier of this important instinct.

I even observe this instinct in my dog, Dallas. She has toys that we call her "stuffies." There is a duck, a moose, a lamb, a palm tree and a couple more animals that she has mangled beyond recognition. She knows that these toys are hers, and to my great satisfaction she chews and grooms only these toys and leaves everything else in the house alone. Sometimes we have other dogs over to visit and they also like her toys. Even though she has multiple toys and can only play with one at a time, whenever other dogs come over, she constantly tries to move *all* her toys away from the other dogs. Instead of rationalizing that "you can have some of my toys, and I will have some of my toys, and we will both be happy playing," she never gives up wanting *all* the toys. I would define this as her instinct for greed, or part of a selfish instinct.

Accepting that selfishness and greed are major motivators of human beings will serve us well as we do our best to navigate our diverse communities, corporate cultures and social structures. In the developed world, our mass media and marketing-enhanced economy have driven a definite focus on a "me first" culture. Social media has given many people the ability to document their daily activities, even rewarding "influencers" who live their lives to excess. The vast majority of "reality" television is driven by outlandish behaviours that can initially be noticed and celebrated on social media, leading to large followings of fans, and then these "characters" are transferred into more traditional entertainment streams with their own television shows, YouTube channels, podcasts or sometimes even cameo appearances in popular films. In most cases, these self-focused, "look at me" behaviours are rewarded with fame, adoration by fans and, in some cases, millions of dollars in financial compensation.

Throughout history we can find thousands of real-life examples of greed in action, and you may have witnessed the instinct for greed ultimately cause the demise of a person involved or "immersed" in this behaviour. It is not flattering to be described as a "greedy" person, and in most civilizations this behaviour and its negative attributes are frowned upon. Greed or selfishness are instincts we need to understand better so that we can control their influence over us. Most of us are taught in kindergarten that "sharing is caring" and, like many of the rules we learn as children, the ability to understand and live these community values can enrich our lives as adults.

The best way to enhance our survival instincts is to gain a better understanding of how they are influencing our actions. Many of these instincts are present at birth and will influence us for most of our life. Our human desires for adequate sleep, food and water form a significant part of these instincts, and it will always serve us well from a survival perspective to try to structure our life so that we are meeting these three basic needs in the best way possible. Acknowledging that we have an instinct for greed that encourages us to always strive for "more" is important too.

TRAINING TIP: Survival Instincts

Most human beings have a basic awareness of their survival instincts; we would not have advanced as a species without them. But it is interesting to note how often we do not meet our basic requirements for sleep, food and hydration. Many of our latest developments and efficiencies as a society have pushed us toward daily habits that leave us under-slept and in many cases over-nourished (with empty calories).

If you think about your survival instincts as representing the bare minimum, this can help you structure a schedule with an enhanced focus on your basic needs. Considering that these are actions you carry out every single day, small changes can make a big impact. You need a basic amount of nutrients each day, a basic amount of hydration and a basic amount of sleep. This "amount" is different for everyone. You may want to consult a professional nutritionist for help determining what exactly "a basic amount" looks like for you. Your nutritional requirements will be based on your height, weight, muscle mass and fat mass along with your daily activity levels. The essential topic of sleep will be discussed in more detail in chapter 12. In all of these areas, knowledge is power, and it helps to clearly understand your basic needs before coming up with a detailed plan for how to meet them.

When it comes to our instincts related to greed and selfishness, things can get much more complicated. The story I related of Dallas always wanting to have "all" of her toys is cute because she is a dog and we find these "human" behaviours in animals entertaining. However, we all know that this behaviour is not so cute when we are talking about adults, and it is more common than we would probably like to admit. Even though we all have strong protective drives related to our own personal situation, human beings for millennia have understood that working as part of a group, tribe or community is more effective than operating as an individual. If we maintain that focus and understand that our connections to other humans also have a positive impact on our overall health, this will help us rationalize our drive away from greed and selfish behaviours and toward a lifestyle that benefits all of humanity.

RECOMMENDED READING: *Sapiens: A Brief History of Humankind* by Yuval Noah Harari

7

Instincts for Animal Connection

I went to the woods because I wished to live deliberately, to front only the essential facts of life, and see if I could not learn what it had to teach, and not, when I came to die, discover that I had not lived.

HENRY DAVID THOREAU, WALDEN

AFTER GIVING BIRTH to our third child, I was trying to figure out a good strategy for getting back to some level of fitness. A few close friends had started a yoga class at a nearby studio and asked if I would be interested in joining them. Exercising with friends is something I always love to do, so I decided to give it a try. I showed up to my first class in an extremely hot studio that was literally packed with people. I soon realized that if you wanted to get a decent spot in this class (for me, that was at the back), you had to show up early! I struggled through my first few classes, but always left feeling great. The instructor, Duncan Parviainen, was wonderful and inspiring. He always made you feel that you had accomplished something amazing simply by showing up and finishing the class. Duncan had a huge following of dedicated yogis, and after a while I noticed that these women who came regularly to his class were doing things at a much higher level of intensity than I had ever imagined in a yoga class. To be fair, this class was called Vinyasa III—one of the higher-level classes.

On the couple of mornings each week when I had no patients scheduled, I could get my kids off to school and then rush to class. The operative word here is "rush." I had to leave extra time for morning traffic and make sure I could battle my way into a parking spot, then basically sprint to the front door of the class. As often happens with young children, things did not always go according to plan. On one extra-busy day, there was way too much crying and complaining and I had that sinking feeling that I was just too late and exhausted to fight for a spot in yoga class. I admitted defeat and walked out the front door into a nearby ravine, thinking that although I would not get a super-intense workout in, I could at least go for a walk.

Everything changed that day. I came back from my walk feeling as though all the troubles and stress from my crazy morning had been lifted away. My brain had a chance to work through a few challenges I was dealing with at work, and at the same time I felt that my body had moved enough that I could consider this outing as exercise. I did make it back to yoga a few times, but soon the allure of the ravine overcame all desire to get into a car, drive through morning traffic, find my yoga mat and water bottle and struggle to find a space in a busy class.

Fast-forward ten years: I rarely miss a day in the ravine, but I probably still have about five yoga classes sitting on my pass at the studio.

As my walks in the ravine continued and my research knowledge grew, I would beg the rest of my family to accompany me on any type of hike, walk or outdoor experience. I would bribe them with things I could buy them while on the hike, such as a doughnut or cookies, or I would use my birthday or Mother's Day as times they should definitely want to come on a hike with me. Now that I have two teenagers in the house, this is becoming more challenging.

One day stands out in my memory. There was no school that day because of parent–teacher interviews and for some reason my daughter was awake early enough and in a good-enough mood that I thought I might tempt her to come along. I said, "If you come on a walk with me, I'll buy you a hot chocolate on the way home." She agreed. We set out along my usual trail and were having a great time. She laughed at me because as I passed some of my regular "hiking friends," I would make a big deal of petting their dogs, almost all of whom I knew by name. After about a mile of walking and about 15 dogs later, my daughter stated, "You know, Mom, it's getting a bit weird with you and all the dogs, it's almost like you are a 'dog stalker'... I think we need to get a dog already!"

At this point in our walk, all the good endorphins were flowing, the trees were embracing us with their beauty and mist, and I thought her statement was absolutely brilliant, so we spent the rest of the walk plotting how we would get Tim to agree that it was time to get a dog. This time in the ravine with my daughter would become a pivotal moment, and it happened at a crucial juncture in my life. I was thinking more about the links between mental health and physical health because of some challenges I was seeing with a couple of my patients. At the same time, I was watching my own children sometimes thriving and sometimes struggling with schedules and demands that seemed a bit extreme. Like all parents, I was doing my best to raise them in the healthiest environment I could provide, but I was not sure the structure we had developed was as good as it could be.

My daughter, with the full support of her two brothers and me, would eventually convince Tim that the arguments for getting a dog were more convincing than anything he could push back at us. In April 2018, we welcomed Dallas, a nine-week-old German shepherd–collie cross, into our lives. Today, I have no idea why we waited so long.

I spent the first few weeks of puppy life slightly sleep deprived but enjoyed every moment of welcoming this adorable creature into our family. The positive energy a puppy brings into a house is indescribable.

Dallas and I made our way into the ravine, rain or shine, almost every day. This was the highlight of my day, and although there were many tear-filled walks, as I was still processing my dad's death, I always felt significantly better when I returned than when I had left. Without her and that time spent in nature, I am sure my recovery would have taken much longer.

Dallas looks remarkably similar to a coyote and is often mistaken for one as she bursts out of the forest toward unsuspecting hikers. Our ravine has several resident coyotes, and owners of small dogs are always on the lookout. One beautiful spring day, as we started up the hill on our way out of the ravine, I looked over just in time to spot three beautiful coyotes on the other side of the creek. It is rare to see more than one, and I soon realized they were probably siblings, because they looked as though they were not quite full-grown. An amazing thing happened that morning. We stopped to watch them because they were playing and wrestling with each other. Their body language and playful behaviours were identical to what I saw from Dallas and her playmates in the ravine. I was completely in awe of the similarities as I realized that, genetically, the coyotes and Dallas were not as far removed as I might think.

As Dallas grew, I was fascinated with how her mannerisms and movements evolved. She became a much better hunter and even managed to catch some of the squirrels she went after. I noticed that this behaviour made her extremely excited and almost joyful as she ran ahead of me on our trail.

Of course, I did not teach her how to hunt small animals; these movements and actions were just a part of her. At certain times of the year, her fur and colouring camouflages her in the leaves and the trees. She hunts using a technique of "sneak" attack that is fascinating to watch. In the winter months, she uses a completely different technique to find mice in the snow. She will listen and smell, then pounce; it almost looks as though she is diving head-first into the snow.

You may be wondering where I am going with all of this, because most of us know that many breeds of dog have hunting instincts. But this instinct was not really the part that interested me as much as what happened after the hunting escapades. I realized that Dallas was much happier after the walks that involved more of her instinctual behaviours, including chasing other dogs and chewing on sticks and grass, and if she came even close to catching a smaller prey, that definitely seemed to be a "mind-blowing" day for her. There were occasional days when we did not make it into the ravine, because my

The subconscious
behaviour of humans
is not as far removed
from that of animals as
we might think.

———————

schedule was too packed. On those days, I had a sad, despondent dog moping around the house.

Living in a large city with an estimated 230,000 dogs (according to the City of Toronto website), I wondered how many of them were able to hunt and run freely in nature. I pictured many dogs who spend a large portion of their day in small apartments, with a couple of walks through a concrete jungle, and I wondered how this affected their overall health and well-being. This type of thinking is not about judging other dog owners and assuming that dogs in apartments are not as happy as dogs running in ravines. In fact, I have met a few breeds of dog that do not enjoy walking in the ravine, dislike bad weather, fear bigger dogs and are incredibly happy with their indoor environment. But I happen to have a dog that is basically the opposite. If we were looking at this through a scientific lens, one might also argue that because she was raised going into the ravine as a puppy, she developed some of those traits and behaviours as a result of her environment.

I believe the subconscious behaviour of humans is not as far removed from that of animals as we might think. Nor are the things that bring us joy, keep us healthy and encourage us to perform at our best. When I watch Dallas and her joyful behaviour outside, I automatically wonder how similar these traits are in humans. I am absolutely convinced that when I am able to get my children to come outside and spend some time running and playing, their mood changes dramatically. It takes a lot of convincing to get them out there, but without fail I am soon hearing laughter and seeing smiling faces. The joy that Dallas expresses when she is able to catch another animal, or play a game of chase with a really fast dog, I think is comparable to how humans feel when we win some type of physical competition such as a race or a football game, or even when we participate in a non-competitive endurance event that challenges us. It is a moment when our basic instinctual abilities are able to outperform the competition or our environment. I am basically saying that something we perceive as a "win" is beneficial to our overall health and well-being. Animals and humans seem to have similar responses to these positive results. Dallas is a huge part of the inspiration for this book, and she helped me study the concept of instincts in real time. Our regular walks, along with time spent observing her daily interactions with nature, are still helping me understand the best way to put all these pieces together.

I do believe that spending time with our pets, or even around wildlife, has both physical and mental health benefits. Animals are used regularly for all types of therapy (dogs, horses and even dolphins). The unconditional love that we receive from a pet can reward us with feelings of contentment and even great joy. A friendship formed with an animal can help alleviate feelings of loneliness and reduce stress. One of the things I find most enjoyable about our dog is that no matter how quickly things change in the world around me, her world, habits, needs and happiness seem to remain exactly the same. Some days the repetitiveness of it can be very calming and almost meditative to me.

The positive benefits of relationships between animals and humans has recently become an important area of health research. Initial findings of studies evaluating the cardiovascular benefits of pet ownership, along with some obvious mental health benefits, included the following:

- Decreased blood pressure
- Decreased levels of cortisol (stress hormone)
- Increased levels of oxytocin (happiness hormone)
- Decreased cholesterol levels
- Decreased triglyceride levels
- Decreased feelings of loneliness
- Increased opportunities for exercise and outdoor activities
- Increased opportunities for socialization

Pet ownership in a city environment is much different from my early life experiences with dogs or barn cats on the farm. In a farming environment, most animals are viewed as "working" pets. Dogs are around for protection and herding, and are basically used as a warning system, to keep unwanted wild animals away. Barn cats were primarily used to control mice and rats. In my current situation, by contrast, I basically work for Dallas: I walk her, I feed her, I take her to the groomer or the vet; she is part of my daily planning as I make sure all her needs are met—not too different from the other members of the family. The good vibes she gives back to all of us make this extra work completely worth it. Our house has become a happier, cuddlier place since Dallas entered it. We do go on more walks together because of her, and to me that fact alone makes having a dog worthwhile.

TRAINING TOOL: Animal Instinct

Get yourself a dog or some other type of pet! I am only half joking here. If you can have a pet in your current situation and are interested in it, I wholeheartedly think this is something worth pursuing, on the understanding that pet ownership is a huge responsibility and that there are significant financial costs associated with it. Remember that although we think of dogs and cats as the most common types of pets for humans, they are not the only options. Research has shown that all types of pets can have positive effects. Fish and turtles can be much easier to manage from a time and cost perspective.

However, if you do not think you could effectively manage having a pet, you should not get one just for the health benefits. In a situation where pet ownership is not suitable to your lifestyle, getting a pet could have the opposite effect, causing you additional stress. If you suspect that you fall into a category where pet ownership would add to your stress, there are better options. You could volunteer to help your friends with their pets, taking them out for an occasional walk or pet-sitting them. There are many shelters for all types of animals and they are always looking for volunteers; this could be a fantastic way to experience the benefits of animal connection without the added responsibility of pet ownership. Even heading to a local park bench with some (environmentally approved) birdseed could become a beautiful routine that would allow you to make some new feathered friends.

If you are already a pet owner, all you need to do now is take a big sigh as you spend time with your beloved animal, knowing that you are improving your health and body chemistry as you do so. How cool is that!

RECOMMENDED READING: *Never Cry Wolf* by Farley Mowat; *The Call of the Wild* by Jack London

8

Instincts for Human Connection

In art as in love, instinct is enough.

ANATOLE FRANCE

ALL HUMAN BEINGS have some brain pathways that are physically present but remain dormant until they are turned on by certain stages of development or possibly certain hormones. A good example of this would be our instinct to reproduce. When we are younger, babies and reproduction are simply a curiosity. Most children find the thought of partnering with another human "disgusting." My kids would always look away or cover their eyes at any love scene that happened to pop up in one of our family movie nights, muttering "So gross!!" until the scene was finished. Boys and girls generally prefer to socialize within their own gender in the early years of their lives—and then puberty hits, and suddenly the world shifts beneath us.

As a parent of teenagers, it has become very obvious to me that the young adults who come storming through our place, devouring massive amounts of food, have quite different ideas about what their social activities should be. The boys who have not yet gone through puberty are incredibly happy to head to the basement and play video games together. At the same time, the boys who are more developed are very interested in heading out for adventures that could involve people other than their close group of friends. They are looking to expand their circle of connections and find more people to socialize with, usually members of the opposite sex. When I overhear these boys negotiating their plans for the night, those who have not reached puberty think the boys who want to go out are basically crazy. "Why would we go out?! We have a PS5. We have food and we are *all* here!" As the frustration levels escalate, you can feel the more "mature" boys already planning their escape.

These behaviours make perfect sense when you understand that, as human beings, we all have basic instincts, or neuronal pathways, that are there to drive certain behaviours. Once we are able to link our behaviours to our instincts, we will start to understand our actions better, and when we realize that certain actions have negative consequences while others have positive outcomes, we then have something better to work with. Our instincts for connection influence many positive and negative behaviours in our everyday lives. Human connection also has a large influence on our overall happiness. Gaining a better understanding of these important instincts allows us to navigate our relationships much more smoothly.

Instincts for Procreation

There is another quite common instinctual situation that may lead to choices that defy logic, especially when we are in our late teenage years and 20s. That is our instinct to find a partner and eventually procreate to ensure our genetic line lives on when we die. I know that, based on the theory of evolution, procreation is always cited as the origin of the original drive, but having witnessed many of these behaviours for over 50 years, I would argue that the hormonal drive behind some of them is not directly linked to the production of offspring. I have never witnessed anyone, male or female, suggest that we should all head over to our friends' party to see how many pregnancies we can cause. I would suggest that there is an extraordinarily strong neural drive to connect with other humans in various ways, and that the drive to produce offspring is a separate matter.

I am sure you have witnessed or possibly even experienced some of the bad decisions human beings can make when our drive is initiated by our instinct to have a physical (most often sexual) connection with another human. Our current media landscape is filled with cases where these very same decisions have led to a sex scandal or legal action. We all probably know someone who has had an affair on their spouse, even though they solemnly swore they would never do such a thing. Lately, we have seen many high-profile men fired and disgraced as a result of the #MeToo movement. More than any other instinct, I feel that the drive for connection can lead to effects that are detrimental or even harmful for the people involved.

But on the flip side, this instinct can also lead to some of the most monumental, positive, life-changing moments. A whole "romance" industry would not exist if it were not for this particularly important instinct to connect and find a partner. Many of the most influential artists of our time will say that they were inspired to greatness by their love for another human being. This instinct and the behaviours, drives or actions that result from it occupy an exceptionally large portion of our lives, making it essential that we try to gain a better understanding of this instinct and how it can alter the trajectory of our life.

These instincts for connection and procreation change significantly throughout a lifetime. Our motivations to connect when we are 18 to 25 years old are often quite different from our motivations to connect when we are 50 or 70. There are vast amounts of excellent research on our need to connect, and new research indicates that the quality of our connections has a direct impact on our health.

The Harvard Study of Adult Development began in 1938 with the ambitious goal of tracking the lives of 268 Harvard sophomores throughout their lives. The goal of the research was initially to uncover clues as to which lifestyle factors would lead to a healthy and happy life. Many health-related variables were studied, and currently (over 80 years later), 19 of the men are still alive, in their mid-90s. This research is important not simply because it represents one of the longest studies of this type ever undertaken; the findings were very surprising to many of the researchers involved. The Harvard men were matched with a cohort of inner-city Boston residents, possibly to evaluate the influence of education and wealth on our overall health, with a hypothesis that the Harvard graduates would lead healthier, happier lives thanks to their higher levels of education. This is not exactly what was determined. The results were so shocking that they have now become a very popular TED Talk by Dr. Robert Waldinger, one of the lead researchers in the current study. The study evaluated these men according to both physiological and mental health variables. The one outstanding finding is described by Waldinger in his TED Talk: "The clearest message that we get from this study is this: Good relationships keep us happier and healthier. Period."

Even though this study evaluated many other factors that we previously suspected would lead to a long and healthy life, including heart and brain health, cardiovascular fitness, socio-economic status, meaningful employment and healthy living conditions, the clear finding was that the quality of our relationships is more important than any of these.

Our society's current fascination with social media and making connections online will probably not produce the positive benefits we are looking for. This research found that the type of relationship was important, as was how close you feel to the people around you. As Waldinger explains: "It's not just the number of friends you have, and it's not whether or not you're in a committed relationship, it's the quality of your close relationships that matters."

These findings are fascinating because when I think about the intense drive that comes from our instinct to connect, I do believe it can lead us down many bad paths, as it often does not guide us toward the high-quality connections mentioned in this research. The divorce rate in most advanced societies is over 50 percent, and this is often accompanied by bad behaviour, selfish actions, diminishing self-worth and even physical and mental abuse. It is striking that an instinct that is so important for our overall health and well-being can also have these negative effects.

Here are a few examples of negative effects arising from our instinct to connect:

- Settling for a partner who you know is not that great for you because you are panicking that you will never find "the right one," so this one will have to do for now

- Showing off by doing ridiculous things, speaking very loudly or dressing in a certain way with the goal of attracting the attention of a potential mate

- Using substances such as alcohol or drugs to alter your state of consciousness so that you are not as nervous when you try to communicate or connect with a potential partner

- Tolerating an emotionally or physically abusive relationship because you feel it is ultimately better than being alone

- Sacrificing your own goals, beliefs or morals in order to follow and support a partner

I observed most of these behaviours in my friends, teammates and colleagues, and sometimes in myself, during my later high school and university years. This makes sense, as these are the prime years for biological reproduction of our species. However, I was not that interested in dating during these years, so when I say I "observed," that is true. I did participate in dating, because that was what I thought was socially acceptable at the time; however, none of my relationships would last much past the four-week mark, when I would start to panic

The quality of our connections has a direct impact on our health.

that my relationship was derailing my other (more important) life goals. I was constantly frustrated as I watched friends fall head over heels for someone and basically drop all other aspects of their life, including spending time with friends. To me it seemed as though their brains had fallen right out of their heads. Looking back on this time, I can probably explain my unorthodox behaviour as a result of delayed hormones that would have triggered a more traditional pattern of dating.

I am now witnessing these same behaviours with friends of my children. The girls they refer to as "boy crazy" are usually the ones who have gone through puberty first, along with the boys who are often classified as "party animals" owing to their loud "look at me" behaviours. It can be helpful to understand these behaviours for what they are: instinctual patterns driven by a strong hormonal desire to connect with another human. It would have been so much easier if I had understood that my friends, teammates and colleagues had not turned into completely different people, but that their hormones were drastically influencing their behaviours in a different way and that my hormones were not on the same timeline.

I noticed a similar pattern of behaviour with my dog the first time she was in heat. Suddenly my happy, confident, playful and somewhat competitive dog had a completely different personality. Every time she came near a male dog that she found attractive, she turned into a "crazy" love dog, doing absolutely everything in her power to try to get the male dog to notice her. In one instance, she was frantically licking one such dog under his chin, and he was obviously not interested in her, and then she proceeded to flop onto her back right in front of him. To the vast amusement of the male dogs' owners, nothing I said or did could get her to stop. I would eventually drag her away from the male dog and sternly tell her, "You are embarrassing yourself and me!" This was not so far removed from conversations I have had with some people!

A Personal Learning about Relationships and Instincts

My training schedule during my first few years of university was intense and demanding. Many days, I would complete two training sessions because I was preparing for the heptathlon. I would work on one event for a couple of hours in the morning and then another in the afternoon. I went through puberty late, at approximately 17 years old, and during all the years of my undergraduate degree I was oligomenorrheic (having infrequent menstruation), possibly because of my intense training schedule. What I did not know at the time but now understand is that my levels of estrogen were extremely low, and my testosterone was probably slightly more elevated than normal owing to the high volume of training.

For some reason, I was also constantly plagued with injuries. One very persistent problem was diagnosed as a stress fracture in my fibula. I went through a year of rehab, cortisone shots, ice baths—you name it, we tried it. Finally, I was sent to an endocrinologist, who assessed that my estrogen was too low and that this could be a possible cause of the stress fractures (in females, estrogen has an impact on bone development). According to the doctors, an easy solution would be for me to go on birth control to increase my levels of estrogen. But because those levels were already so low, the first pill basically caused me to have an emotional meltdown. I would cry daily for no reason. My energy levels were often too low for me to train, and I knew this could not be a long-term solution to my problem.

Many months later, we were able to adjust the dosage, and I was placed in a cast to heal the fracture. My competitive athletics career never returned to pre-injury levels, but at the same time I was doing well at school, finishing my master of science degree, and I had started dating someone who, for some reason, I still really liked even after my usual four-week cut-off point. I am not suggesting that the increased estrogen levels in my system triggered an instinctual drive to find a partner, but in retrospect, I am sure the timing was not entirely coincidental.

Tim, among his many amazing talents and attributes, loves spending time in nature. As described earlier, I had shunned the forests and woods for life in the thriving metropolis of Saskatoon. Any time I had a chance to travel, I would seek out larger cities, because that was what I found exciting. Things were different with Tim. Much of our time together was spent on long walks through various trails in the city, eventually leading to camping trips, ski trips to the mountains and spending days and weeks exploring northern Saskatchewan. Eventually, I decided that Tim and I should head to the farm so he could see what my life there was like and to spend some time with my dad. It was no surprise that Tim loved the farm and my dad. He came with us on our hiking expeditions, and my dad took him trap shooting (although I made it very clear that Tim should never shoot a live animal). He helped my dad during many harvests, and he even brought his own parents out during harvest time, so they could experience this beautiful place that was very influential in the early years of our relationship.

As much as we loved our time at the farm, we knew how hard it would be to make a living with the price of wheat very low. We both had great jobs in Saskatoon, so we never considered that we would live in a rural community. One of Tim's many positive influences on my life was to return me to my love of nature, and I am forever grateful for that. However, our jobs were dependent on universities and research, so we slowly made our way east. We eventually landed in Toronto and were married that same fall. We were both working at the University of Toronto. I was a sessional lecturer for a class called Research Design and Statistics, while Tim was working in the biomechanics lab and as a server at the Bloor Street Diner on the side.

Our usual trips to relax in nature diminished during these years. Our lives were fairly good, extremely busy, while at the same time incredibly productive. The one thing we both knew how to do was work extremely hard. We moved to Toronto knowing absolutely no one. We had no family or friends, and basically no community to support us. Having left a small city where it felt as if we knew almost everyone, and where we had probably benefited from a bit of the "big fish in a small pond" situation, we felt out of our element in Toronto. Externally, we presented ourselves as confident, capable and hard-working individuals, but at the same time we were basically working constantly to prove ourselves in this completely new environment.

We spent more time arguing, and we suffered hugely from the effects of increased negative stress in our lives, with no healthy way to alleviate it. We were working hard and playing hard in a city with no downtime. Our lives were consumed with long hours of work followed by tons of social activities, because we were meeting so many new people every day and trying to form friendships. Although many of these same people are now very good friends, at this point they were mostly acquaintances, and if you remember from the Harvard men's study, it is very deep relationships that are the most beneficial to your health. We did not have this type of relationship yet with anyone in Toronto.

Weeks turned into months, and as time flew by, there was no chance to slow down, take a break or reassess our lifestyle choices. Every day brought new challenges or adventures, and our intense behaviours continued. Eventually, our relationship started to break down. At the end of the next summer we decided that our fighting and arguments had progressed to the level where we could no longer be together. Tim found himself a rental unit in a boarding house and moved out. We felt like total failures, who were possibly not even going to make it through one full year of marriage. I had been hospitalized twice for major strep infections that could only be cured through IV antibiotics. Our lifestyle, with its constant stress and lack of downtime, was destroying both our health and our relationship.

Tim left Toronto late that summer to help my dad with the harvest. At that time, I was convinced we would be heading straight toward a divorce when he returned. Approximately one month later, he showed up at Toronto General Hospital to help me through one of the worst strep infections of my life (my third hospitalization), followed by a major surgery to remove my chronically infected tonsils. Even though we were both working out regularly and eating well, we were missing something crucial in our current situation. My energy levels were at an all-time low; it took me an exceptionally long time to completely recover from the surgery, and I knew something had to drastically change if I was going to continue living and working in Toronto.

Tim came back from the farm a different person. Through counselling, we developed strategies to help us work on our relationship challenges. Consequently, we both started spending way more time outdoors, and began coaching some of our clients for marathons. I would walk home from work most days, and Tim bought a bike that he rode almost daily. The stress in our lives did not actually decrease during this time, but as we explored the trails through Toronto and realized that even one night spent in the beautiful countryside outside the city was enormously helpful to our overall well-being, we became happier and much healthier.

Instincts and Attraction

Why are we attracted to certain things or people and not others? There are instinctual explanations for some of these attractions. Many of our physical characteristics developed through evolution over thousands of years, influenced by our landscapes and environments. If your tribe lived close to the equator in an extremely hot climate, having more melatonin in your skin tone would protect you from the damaging effects of sun exposure. If you lived in an

In our current century, instincts that drive attraction are possibly becoming more diverse when compared with previous centuries.

———————

extremely cold climate, having a darker skin tone was no advantage, but an extra layer of body fat would help you survive in colder temperatures. Survival meant that your genetic characteristics would be passed on to a new generation. Those people who did not have physical attributes suited to the climate would be less likely to survive, and therefore their genetics would not continue to the next generation. In a general sense, we are attracted to potential mates who appear to have strong genes, and who we think are healthy, with a likelihood of surviving as long as we will. There are more complicated theories which suggest that women are more attracted to men who appear strong and athletic, and that men are attracted to women who seem fertile. In our current century, because many of the boundaries related to travel and migration are dissolving, instincts that drive attraction are possibly becoming more diverse when compared with previous centuries.

A world-renowned researcher in social psychology, Donn Byrne was most famous for his theories on similarity and attraction between human beings. The oft-quoted phrase "birds of a feather flock together" was scientifically verified throughout his four decades of groundbreaking research in this area. When studying a group comprising hundreds of college-aged students, Byrne found that the only significant determinant of attraction was similarity, even though several other variables were measured.

For many decades, the Federal Bureau of Investigation (FBI) has used these psychological theories as part of their hostage negotiation protocols. One of their most famous and successful negotiators, Chris Voss, has gone on to teach a master class on this very subject. In his recent bestselling book about the topic, *Never Split the Difference*, Voss explains the concept of mirroring in more detail:

Mirroring, also called isopraxism, is essentially imitation. It's another neurobehavior humans (and other animals) display in which we copy each other to comfort each other. It can be done with speech patterns, body language, vocabulary, tempo, and tone of voice. It's generally an unconscious behavior—we are rarely aware of it when it is happening—but it's a sign that people are bonding, in sync, and establishing the kind of rapport that leads to trust.

It makes sense that this behaviour would be extremely helpful in a high-stress negotiation, and Voss goes on to explain why it works: "It's a phenomenon (and now a technique) that follows a very basic but profound biological principle: We fear what is different and are drawn to what is similar."

When I think of these "laws of attraction" and how they might apply to an everyday situation, I realize that I am personally interested in, or drawn to, people who I think have similar beliefs, interests and hobbies as me, and I am sure that is why social media engines such as Facebook have a large portion of the platform dedicated to "likes." Whether we "like" this idea or not, once we engage with these platforms, our interests, political beliefs and even choices of music are constantly being analyzed and then grouped into various levels of marketing strategies.

When we understand this instinct of attraction, we can control its influence over our behaviour much more effectively. If we know that we are automatically drawn to or attracted by things and people we think are like us, we can then logically decide if our instinct is correct in each case. Similarly, if we know that something quite different from ourselves may initially cause a reaction of fear or hesitation, we should use our cognitive analysis to determine if this fear is warranted. In many cases, it could unconsciously cause us to avoid things that we might enjoy, and which might present an opportunity for expanding our understanding of something we are not familiar with.

TRAINING TOOL: Instincts for Human Connection

Positive and lasting human connections are one of the essential determinants of our overall health and happiness. In the corporate world, you could also argue that they are extremely important for success. Understanding how our instinctual patterns drive our behaviours related to relationships and connection should help us form better, longer-lasting bonds with other human beings. At the same time, knowing how important these connections are, we must realize that dedicated effort is required to initiate relationships and maintain them. For so many reasons, these extra efforts will be beneficial to our overall well-being and are worth the extra introspection and understanding required to honour our basic instincts.

Accepting that many of the behaviours related to human connection are driven by our hormones can allow us insight into these behaviours when they occur at various periods of our own and others' development. Many parents instinctively understand that some days we need to give our teenagers a "pass" on some of the seemingly ridiculous things they do or say, because we know this is a period of life when hormones are turning on pathways the teen does not yet fully understand. It is also natural for their hormones to push them away from their parents both emotionally and physically, because this is the time for them to acquire their independence. Having open and supportive conversations about these things as a family can go a long way to preserving everyone's sanity during these challenging years of development.

After spending months in isolation during the 2020 pandemic, we have all probably gained a new and profound appreciation of the importance of human connection. There were literally hundreds of strategies coming from all over the world, presented on our screens in a regular rotation: neighbours in lawn chairs talking across a street, people singing on balconies, Zoom drinks, FaceTime everything. I am sure you noticed an overall increased level of daily stress because of your limited ability to interact with friends and family. I cannot imagine the levels of despair experienced by our seniors living in long-term-care homes, who were suddenly cut off from the rest of the world. It has been a lesson for all of humanity that should never be forgotten and hopefully will never be repeated.

RECOMMENDED READING: *Never Split the Difference: Negotiating as if Your Life Depended on It* by Chris Voss

9

Instincts and Family Life

Instinct is a marvellous thing.
It can neither be explained nor ignored.

AGATHA CHRISTIE,
THE MYSTERIOUS AFFAIR AT STYLES

WHEN I WAS around 25 years old, if you had asked me, "Do you think you will get married and start a family?" I would probably have answered you with a hard "No!" Having grown up in a traditional farming family, I was adamant that a lifestyle of raising children, gardening, and cooking and cleaning for men who were at work all day was absolutely not for me. At a young age I quickly recognized that the men who worked in the fields were treated like "kings" while the women who worked at home were not referred to or valued as the equivalent "queens." I have vivid memories of my mom sitting on the kitchen floor in tears as the stress of getting a huge meal out to the field during harvest time became overwhelming. My brother and I would fight over who got to work with my dad and who had to stay home to help around the house. One day you would be treated as an essential force of productivity and praised for your efforts, the next day as though your work did not even exist.

I was proud that I had managed to become a successful, independent female working in a science field dominated by men, and I was thriving both financially and intellectually. Having children was not part of that picture, in my opinion. I dreaded being invited to my friends' baby showers; I did not even know how to hold a baby because I had no interest in babysitting, ever! I mostly viewed pregnancy and motherhood as modern society's evil strategy to prevent women from reaching their full potential. I had read Margaret Atwood many times, and I did not feel that some of the concepts alluded to in *The Handmaid's Tale* were too far-fetched.

Even after almost a decade of married life, I was holding on to these beliefs quite strongly. Tim and I were one of the few couples in our social circles who had not decided to have children. We had travelled the world, spending months exploring Europe, Asia and the United States. I was travelling to academic conferences in other countries to present my research findings. In my field, I felt that I could hold my own in any debate with the best and the brightest. As I have described in previous chapters, we certainly knew how to work hard and play hard. Our social calendars were constantly booked with fun and entertaining events, shared with great friends.

One night, after returning from a wonderful trip to the south of France, we found ourselves at a party that occurred annually as part of the Toronto International Film Festival. We had managed to secure an invite to the VIP section of the *Vanity Fair* party. We were surrounded by celebrities, and the paparazzi were out in full force, with constant flashes going off in every direction. There had been much anticipation about this particular party because of who was supposed to be in attendance, and we were excited to be caught up in the frenzy. A couple of hours and three or four (watered-down) cocktails into the party, I looked at Tim and said, "Are you as bored as I am with all this?" He sighed and said, "I knew you were excited about this party, so I didn't want to say anything... but I am SO bored!" We made a discreet exit and hopped into a cab to be dropped off at our favourite late night restaurant, 7 West Cafe.

I am not sure if there is an instinctual reason why food always tastes better when you are drinking very late at night, but it always does. (Possibly part of our survival instincts, probably directly related to alcohol consumption and dehydration!) That night, as we relaxed, ate and debriefed about the party, we both decided that we had travelled enough and partied enough to last us for a long time. We also decided that having children was something we would like to commit to.

Less than one year later, our son Matthew was born. Today, those parties and carefree days of travelling without children feel like a lifetime ago, but we have absolutely no regrets.

Maternal and Paternal Instincts

We can regularly observe maternal and paternal instinctual patterns in both humans and animals. These instincts are another good example of pathways that lie dormant in both humans and animals until they are stimulated or turned on, usually by a baby.

The well-researched "feel-good" hormone oxytocin has been demonstrated to have a significant impact on our feelings toward all offspring. An interesting study looked at the effects of oxytocin on mice at various stages of their lifespan. The researchers compared two groups of mice—female virgins and female mothers. Both groups were subjected to crying baby mice. The female virgins would either ignore the babies or, in some cases, cannibalize them(!), whereas the female mothers would search out the crying baby mice and care for them. The researchers then injected the virgin, cannibalizing mice with oxytocin. These mice then searched out the crying pups and cared for them in the same way the female mother mice had, which marked an extremely drastic change in behaviour because of a shift in hormones. This is a great example of how an instinctual pathway can lie dormant and then suddenly be turned on. How did the virgin mice know how to "take care" of the baby mice? It is possibly (probably) an instinctual pattern they were born with. The researchers then went one step further and injected male mice with the hormone. The response was similar. The male mice took longer to notice the young pups crying, but eventually they did retrieve them in a way that resembled the female mice's behaviour.

An instinctual pathway can lie dormant and then suddenly be turned on.

Our society has evolved in many positive ways, with men now participating in many child-rearing responsibilities. Some of the research related to parenting instincts finds a positive shift in levels of oxytocin after exposure to a baby. Females will experience this important hormonal change almost immediately after giving birth, while males experience the same effect once they have a long-enough exposure to a baby.

Instincts and Family Dynamics

As a new parent, I was overwhelmed by the insane amount of advice, books, research, myths, television shows, podcasts, reality shows and even completely unsolicited advice (or praise) from strangers on how best to raise our children. I am not saying this is all negative, but when you are a new parent, it can be daunting. I believe that, because Tim and I chose to have children much later (I was 36, 38 and 40 when I gave birth), we had the life experience and fortitude to be a little more laid-back than we probably would have been in our early 20s. We both worked full-time during these years, and I honestly think that helped us be more efficient when deciding what things to focus on as new parents.

I remember a feeling of exhaustion when I returned to work following my third maternity leave. We had a four-year-old son, a two-year-old daughter and a six-month-old son at home. I would go to work in the morning, then rush home at lunch to breast-feed the baby, quickly grab something to eat and head back to work. I am sure many houses with small children have experienced a similar schedule. Every day of the week, the schedule was basically the same: wake up, have breakfast, engage in morning activities until around 1 p.m.— nap time. By that time, the little ones have been busy all morning with their various outings, play dates and errands, and then they sit down to lunch. Suddenly the house becomes noticeably quiet, you see droopy eyelids, and you know it is time. If you miss this important window, then you enter "overtired" mode, when your cute, sweet toddler who seemed happy only minutes ago seemingly becomes possessed by some evil spirit. It is essential to read the cues and get them into bed before it is too late.

We were extremely fortunate to have a wonderful caregiver at our house during these early years. Floridel "Flor" Elyado was a crucial part of our highly active family. I would not have survived (either mentally or physically) without her. Most parents will agree that during these early years with a baby or toddler at home, your body is running on fumes and adrenalin. I was no exception. When I came home at lunchtime and the house had started to enter nap time, that rare moment of calm, my brain craved sleep. I am quite sure that, instinctually, at this quiet, sleepy time, my body was giving me *very* strong signals that I should be having a nap along with the children. Instead, I would drink some ridiculously strong coffee, hop back into my car, blast the radio and try my best to fight those feelings of fatigue so I could get back to work.

I can honestly say that those years are now a complete blur. Raising young kids, like being in university and athletics, was another great example of my very diminished level of effectiveness as I tried to rally against my biology and basic instincts for rest and sleep.

I was never hard on myself during my pregnancies, worrying what I looked like. As a person who works in health and wellness, I had met many pregnant women as patients and clients who were in a complete panic about the weight they were gaining and struggled to stay fit while they were pregnant. I knew this would not be the case with me; my goals with training are always more driven by performance and how I feel, rather than by what I look like. With my first pregnancy I gained 80 pounds and delivered a 10-pound baby (via C-section). Coming home with a healthy baby was my only goal, and I felt extremely fortunate that I was able to accomplish that. I did not gain quite as much weight with the second two pregnancies, but close. I had been pregnant three times in six years and that had taken a huge toll on all aspects of my life, while at the same time greatly diminishing my overall fitness. I was weaker, my core was literally ripped to pieces (with a huge rectus diastasis), my cardiovascular capacity was non-existent, and so was my ability to mentally push myself through any level of physical discomfort. I felt that I could manage to take care of my family (with lots of help from Flor and Tim) and get myself to work—and that was about it.

Looking back on this sometimes insanely busy time, I am not sure what I would do differently. I know that I benefited tremendously from the help of others, and when I meet or hear about single working parents trying to do the same thing, I honestly have no idea how they survive. What I have observed is that maternal and paternal instincts are possibly some of the most powerful motivators we have as human beings. In the animal world, we see this as well. As a person who hikes regularly, I know that spring is a much more treacherous season if you are hiking anywhere near bear territory. All the analogies of "momma bear" and "do not mess with my cubs" can quickly become an actual life-threatening event if you find yourself face to face with this scary situation.

In humans, it can be helpful to understand the incredibly strong feelings these instincts evoke. We have all heard stories, or possibly even experienced incidents, where parents have gone completely berserk in order to protect or defend their children. Fortunately, in modern society this does not usually happen in a life-threatening situation; instead, it is much more likely to play out in a hockey arena or on the rickety stands of a football field. It is helpful to recognize that these inner feelings can drive your brain to think that *your* child is the smartest, the fastest, the cutest and generally just heads above the others *before* you even enter any of these arenas. This same thinking can then take over in conversations with teachers, coaches and possibly even other parents. I believe that so many conflicts could be resolved much more easily, and that many children would greatly benefit, if all parents acknowledged this instinct and worked to manage their behaviours associated with it. If we realize that this instinct developed for actual life-threatening situations, where the lives of our offspring are legitimately imperilled, we can understand that it should only be acted upon at those times. If you encounter a situation in real life where this is the case, this instinct will serve you well. But it is not often appropriately used in non-life-threatening situations. Please proceed with caution!

TRAINING TOOL: Instincts and Family Life

Remember that the lifestyles we may have created in order to succeed in an often busy or stressful environment are not necessarily the best way to live when it comes to our overall health and happiness. The human body for millennia functioned in unique rhythms linked to the natural environment. It is important to recognize these rhythms and how they affect our family units today. There are many important moments that occur every day within a family or between spouses, but often we are so busy rushing through our daily routines and taking each other for granted that we don't even notice them. These moments can create our best memories of our lives spent with others, but sometimes we need to slow down in order to enjoy them.

RECOMMENDED READING: *In Praise of Idleness* by Bertrand Russell; *Rest, Play, Grow: Making Sense of Preschoolers (Or Anyone Who Acts Like One)* by Dr. Deborah MacNamara

10

Instincts for Communication

*Only through communication
can human life hold meaning.*

PAULO FREIRE

BABIES INHERENTLY KNOW how to cry or otherwise let us know they are uncomfortable, and they develop techniques of communication to get their needs met at a young age. The instinctual human development of speech and language has been well studied for centuries. Like other pathways in our brain, our region of speech has been mapped out, and there are vast amounts of scientific investigation focused on this area of human development. With similar patterns to animals, human beings have instinctual abilities related to the development of communication. Animals do not need to be exposed to sound or imitate sounds to communicate effectively with their species; however, humans have more specific requirements to ensure we develop our ability to communicate effectively. Humans also have a specific window where they are able to access their neural pathways for speech, and as with some of our instinctual movement patterns, once the window has passed, if we miss it, these skills will never develop to their full potential. This critical period is scientifically defined as "a restricted developmental period during which the nervous system is particularly sensitive to the effects of experience." In human beings, this critical period seems to be before puberty. Research in children who are deaf also demonstrates a critical window for learning sign language as a replacement for verbal talking, with a similar time frame. Case studies have shown that in rare cases where children were not exposed to communication prior to puberty, they were not able to regain an ability to speak even after they were transferred to an environment where people attempted to teach them to speak. Speech and communication are great examples of instincts that are turned on at a specific period of our development, and it is important we are aware of this if we want to develop this instinct to its fullest potential.

My interest in human movement is logical, based on what I do in my practice every day. Lately, though, I have realized that effective communication is just as important to what I do. I spend a large part of my treatment time with patients explaining scientific terms, breaking down human movements and, most importantly, trying to motivate people to be healthier. I have encountered and worked with many types of professionals with similar goals to mine. I have observed many techniques of communication first-hand, and I feel that in science and medicine we seriously underestimate the importance of *how* we communicate to our clients and patients, because we are more interested in figuring out the exact problem, tricky diagnosis or, often, in my case, orthopaedic challenge we are dealing with.

I would argue that humans prefer to learn and communicate through stories. Religion is a great example of this. The Bible could simply have been written as a set of rules one must follow to demonstrate your devotion to God. Instead, across the many books of the Bible, we find a series of detailed stories that use various extreme situations and sometimes very dramatic descriptions to help the reader understand and be motivated to follow the dogma or rules of the religion. You can look at almost any religion and you will find the same pattern of lessons, ideas and even rules of behaviour taught through stories. One that stands out is the story that forms the basis of the religion Scientology. In this religion it is believed that approximately 75 million years ago, trillions of aliens were banished to Earth. To make their situation even worse, they were dropped into volcanoes and then apparently vaporized with nuclear bombs. I recall watching this story in an animated version in the movie *Going Clear: Scientology and the Prison of Belief*. Those images are not easy to forget, and this story had a much bigger impact on my ability to remember how Scientology was formed than if someone had simply told me about the structure of the religion. Most people realize that religious stories are not factual or even historical, but the repetition of them, within the massive architectural structures built to host spiritual readings or sermons that bring together the emotionally devoted followers in every community, tends to eventually make these stories as believable as scientific facts to some followers. If only I could figure out a way to turn my patients' exercise prescriptions into something as compelling as aliens falling into volcanoes, I am sure I would have a much better adherence and recollection rate.

Scientists working in the field of climate change have faced massive challenges over the years trying to convince our civilizations that human pollution and industrialization are having a negative effect on the planet. The information related to climate change is most commonly presented to us as a series of scientific discoveries. One exception would be the documentary by Al Gore entitled *An Inconvenient Truth*. This movie finally portrayed climate change as more of a story, with dramatic images and predictions. As a result, the film resonated with millions of people. It had a much larger impact when compared with our regular science reporting of climate change developments. On the other side, the stories that form the basis of many religions are so compelling that there still exist millions of people who do not believe that climate change is real and millions more who believe in a God who will ultimately dictate what happens to our planet.

Many of the best public speakers throughout history used stories to inspire crowds of people. When I listen to my TED Talks podcast, most of the extremely popular speakers have figured out a way to turn

As listeners, we quickly develop a connection to the emotion provided in a story. We have better recall when we have an emotional reaction to what we are being taught.

———————

their topic into a story. As listeners, we quickly develop a connection to the emotion provided in a story. We have better recall when we have an emotional reaction to what we are being taught.

Researchers often discuss interesting problems or findings through the lens of individual case studies. Having read about a wide variety of case studies over many years, along with equally as many double-blind randomized control trials (RCTs), I am sure most scientists would agree that they have better recall and maybe even understanding when they think about unique case studies as opposed to RCT research.

Another interesting aspect of our instincts related to connection and communication is that we respond more intensely to stories that scare us or are about things we are afraid of. These reactions can probably be traced back to our early tribal days, when negative stories were about things that were a real and immediate threat to our existence. These stories would have a much greater level of urgency attached to them because they contained information that could affect the survival of the tribe. You can imagine being approached by someone in your immediate friend or family group who informs you they have specific information about an imminent attack on your family from a warring tribe that is hoping to take over all your hunting territory. This type of news would probably travel quickly through your community because your lives depend on it. Fast-forward to current times, where every successful news organization is hyper-aware of this basic human instinct, to the point where most of our headlines are "sensationalized" into stories that appear to be more threatening than they actually turn out to be. In an hour-long news broadcast, most days will see much of the focus on things that are scary or possibly challenging to human survival. These savvy networks know that, from an instinctual viewpoint, human beings have a challenging time ignoring news that we view as a possible threat to our existence.

Using Effective Communication
to Alter Instinctual Behaviours

Many of our most amazing scientific discoveries were made by people who managed to devote their whole lives to the immersive study of one small aspect of what they were interested in. Today, we often see and hear scientists on our televisions and computers and smartphones, and I am sure you will agree that they are not often as compelling as the actors and entertainers we watch on these very same devices. Remember that humans do have an instinctive drive to connect, and we are always looking for other humans to connect to, whether it be as a fan of a certain performer, or falling in love with a particular actor, or even becoming obsessed with a particular athlete or team. Actors and other performers are aware that their ability to connect with their audience, and in many cases their need to do so, is what drives their success.

The best scientists in the world are probably not overly concerned about how you reacted to their television interview, and this is where some of the facts can get lost in the constant media noise. When big brands are launching a new product that has been recently developed in one of their nutrition or cosmetics labs, one of the first things they do is try to find a compelling spokesperson to represent the brand. If they can afford a celebrity, this is even better. I have been hired to be this person (by companies that did not have the budget for an actual celebrity) for various brands related to the work I do in television. From my point of view, it would be interesting to hear from the scientist who actually invented the new product, but these savvy companies know that in order to sell a product, they need to drive a deep connection to their audience, and usually actors or at least people who regularly work in the media are better at this. Even more importantly in some instances, for example in the case of a product that has scientifically been shown *not* to be good for people but which you are trying to convince them is okay, you need someone with a mesmerizing quality, so that while the audience is in the process of "connecting," they are actually ignoring the facts. We witnessed this years ago with cigarette companies. They sought out people from all areas of life—actors, doctors, even athletes—to try to convince us that smoking was good for our health. We have also seen this phenomenon at the many rallies organized by former president Donald Trump. The audience cheers constantly because of their emotional connection to what he is saying, and as a person very experienced in television, he knows how to communicate with stories, drama, scare tactics and emotion to build on these reactions from his base. The people attending these rallies are not concerned with the facts; they love how the words make them feel emotionally.

A fascinating discovery that sheds light on this concept emerged from several neurological studies, where researchers were able to evaluate various patients and their memories of certain events that had occurred in their life. These events were recorded, and in a subsequent meeting the researchers altered some of the facts, sometimes to the opposite of what had actually happened, and repeatedly reviewed the new "revised" stories with the patients. Eventually, the new stories with the opposite facts became the patients' memories. If you recall the image of our brain as a series of grooved neurological pathways, it is interesting to speculate that these brilliant researchers simply grooved new pathways for their subjects. Once the new pathways became more prominent than the previous ones, they became the subjects' "new" truth.

Understanding that our memories and perception of "facts" can be altered if we hear a different story enough times can be shocking, but I suspect you can find examples of this in your own life. We have all heard the term "pathological liar," and this type of experiment illustrates that our memories are probably not as accurate as we think, and are susceptible to change. It also helps to explain how logical people can make choices and undertake actions that seem to make no sense when observed from a rational, factual or scientific view.

A particularly good example of this happened within our immediate family when our parents died. In a span of four years, we attended the funerals of three parents: my father-in-law, then my mother-in-law, and shortly afterwards my dad. Our children were between the ages of eight and twelve, and we had many interesting discussions about the religious concept of "heaven" related to what exactly their grandparents were doing now that they were no longer with us. Obviously, our kids are well educated in science, and Tim and I are both trained and educated and fully believe in the theory of evolution, but for our children, the story of heaven was much easier to process and visualize as a place where their grandparents were now "resting." All three of the funeral ceremonies had featured people repeatedly speaking about heaven, and many conversations surrounding the funeral also included these ideas. Soon the idea of heaven became a truth for our children. Tim and I did not argue with this choice, but we also did not say that we believed in the concept of heaven, because we do not. We simply told them that they should feel truly fortunate to live in a country (and with a family) where they were able to choose what they wanted to believe about their grandparents, and we were all happy with that.

Instincts for Leadership, Learning and Inspiration

Effective communication has a profound influence on the way we choose various types of leaders in our current society. The previous examples about religion demonstrate how human beings can be emotionally drawn to certain styles of leadership. It is as though our species has an instinctual longing or desire to find inspiration and guidance that will enhance our everyday experiences. Once they

An understanding
of the instinctual patterns
that inspire humans
to communicate, learn and
possibly lead will always
be beneficial to you.

———————

decide what or who will lead them, humans can be so overcome by feelings of "service" or "dedication" that they would willingly die for the person or cause they believe in. Most of us are aware that the phrase "drinking the Kool-Aid" comes from a particularly tragic event that could equally be used to illustrate the term "blind faith." Jim Jones was an extremely charismatic cult leader of a group called the Peoples Temple, originally based in California. He soon grew his following to various locations throughout the United States and a rural compound in Jonestown, Guyana. Following a thorough investigation of the Jonestown commune that resulted in the murders of several government officials, in 1978 Jim Jones ordered his followers to commit suicide by drinking a type of cyanide poisoning mixed with a fruit drink (the Kool-Aid). This unfathomable event resulted in the deaths of over 900 people, including many babies and children. It was a tragic reminder of just how devastating the impacts and decisions of our beloved leaders can be.

I imagine that human leadership in prehistoric times was similar to what we see in animals. The strongest, fastest, most experienced and most aggressive became the natural leaders of a group or tribe. Their ability to hunt and survive various threats better than the rest of the group meant that they were obvious choices to be leaders. Human beings often look for efficiencies as they try to find ways to survive and thrive. I suspect that our search for good leadership is partially related to this desire to be as efficient as possible. We hope that if we join a company with a great leader, we will ride the wave of success together. Similarly, if we decide to move to a country because we are inspired by its leader, we probably believe it offers the best living situation for ourselves and our family. Great leaders throughout history have been notable for their ability to get the most out of their followers. Some of the common techniques or strategies can be traced back to our previous discussions on human motivation. We know that humans can accomplish phenomenal things when we group together, in most cases much more than we could do as individuals. You can probably remember times when you were personally motivated by an individual or a movement that stirred you to perform beyond your usual abilities. We can even experience this phenomenon in something as simple as an exercise class. One of the main reasons people choose to participate in a class is that they know they will be able to push themselves harder when they are part of a group, being led by someone who inspires them . . . or sometimes even scares them!

Throughout history we can find many examples of inspiring leadership that allowed populations to accomplish amazing feats. One leader who springs to mind is Winston Churchill during World War II. His speeches inspired his country and the entire Allied movement to keep going through almost impossible stress, widespread casualties and a massive death toll. Many quotes from his speeches at that crucial time are still repeated today:

If you're going through hell, keep going. Never, never give up.

Success is not final, failure is not fatal—it is the courage to continue that counts.

To improve is to change, so to be perfect is to have changed often.

Courage is what it takes to stand up and speak. Courage is also what it takes to sit down and listen.

It does not matter if you aspire to be the next leader of the free world or would like to find better ways to talk with your teenaged daughter, your co-workers, your partner or your spouse: communication is a skill that can be developed. An understanding of the instinctual patterns that inspire humans to communicate, learn and possibly lead will always be beneficial to you and everyone you connect with.

TRAINING TOOL: Instincts for Communication

Understanding that we have all developed instincts and skills for effective communication will help us find ways to become even better communicators. Maybe your job requires you to motivate a team or speak in public, or maybe you are a coach trying to inspire a group of young athletes. Whatever position you find yourself in, skills for effective communication can always be improved. It is important to recognize that, as with many of our instinctual patterns, there is a critical window where we should strive to optimize our skills for communication. Learning a new language is much easier for human beings before they reach puberty. The challenges will be greater if we try to do this later in life, but it is always possible to improve.

Humans respond best to information told to them in the form of stories. If your story can include an emotional component, such as humour, joy, fear or empathy, it will be more powerful for your audience.

Remember that our memories are not as accurate as we might want to believe. You could test this theory out by asking a friend to recall a shared experience from many years ago. Ask them to explain as many details as possible, then compare those memories with your own. If you try this in a fun, relaxed way, you might find that you and your friends all learn something new and important about how you recall certain events.

Finally, beware the snake oil salesperson! We are surrounded by these people in our current environment. Never-ending news cycles, social media feeds, and the societal challenge of widespread loneliness and depression sometimes create a situation where the loudest voices fill the much-needed quiet times in our lives. Our instinctual patterns can make us more susceptible to fear mongering, slick marketing campaigns or even repeated non-factual statements. Now that you are aware of these challenges, you will be better able to tune out the negative messages and focus on the communications and connections that enhance your well-being.

RECOMMENDED READING: *Talking to Strangers: What We Should Know about the People We Don't Know* by Malcolm Gladwell

RECOMMENDED VIEWING: *An Inconvenient Truth* with Al Gore

11

11

Enhancing and Honouring Our Basic Instincts by Spending More Time in Nature

It was a voice which spoke of the lost world which once was ours before we chose the alien role; a world which I had glimpsed and almost entered . . . only to be excluded, at the end, by my own self.

FARLEY MOWAT, *NEVER CRY WOLF*

I RECALL READING Farley Mowat's *Never Cry Wolf* as a teenager, and I am pretty sure I completely ignored the real premise of the story and simply focused on the "cool" idea of living with wolves, a fantastic concept to me at that time. As I read this quote today, it brings tears to my eyes as I picture a wolf howling because its family members have been killed by humans. More importantly, I feel the sadness attached to the idea of a "lost world" that, at the time Mowat's book was published, was not an actual threat but is now something many of us feel almost daily as a result of our current environmental crisis. Mowat writes about feeling helpless when he discovers that it is not the wolves that are the problem but the humans with their barbaric killing practices. In the end he expresses his frustration as he realizes that even his enlightening discovery after living with the wolves for many months will not result in any meaningful change.

Like most of our human population, I have spent the majority of my life living in larger city centres and often taking nature for granted. As I explained in previous chapters, my attitude shifted when I started dating my now-husband and then was further enhanced by my daily walks in a nearby ravine. The positive benefits I gain from these walks reach far beyond any physiological explanation related to the exercise I am getting.

I have been going into the ravine regularly for approximately five years. Over this time, I cannot recall being sick with a common cold or flu. I have not had to miss a single day of work because of illness. The majority of my health habits have not changed significantly since my early years in Toronto; in fact, I probably get less exercise now and spend more time sitting, owing to demands of work and raising three very active children (I currently spend *way* too much time driving them to various activities). My nutrition is basically the same as when we first moved to Toronto, and my sleep habits are similar—possibly fewer late nights out, compared with before we had children, and we rarely get to sleep in past 9 a.m. anymore. When I think about how I feel today and remember what my life was like when I first moved to Toronto, I am amazed at how much better I feel overall.

Being a person who works in health and fitness, and is obsessed with science and research, as I was returning from my walks I would often wonder why they made me feel so good and why I would guard this precious ravine time in my busy schedule to ensure I could always fit it in. I started to investigate these feelings a bit further to try to understand why my walks in nature left me feeling better than any other workout I tried.

I discovered that I was not imagining the benefits; they were scientifically verifiable. There are many research studies supporting the premise that human beings respond very well to time spent in nature. It is also well understood that trees provide healing and immunity-boosting chemicals to their surrounding areas, including the animals and any humans who happen to be strolling in their midst.

After my husband bought me *The Hidden Life of Trees* by Peter Wohlleben, my daily walks became even more interesting. I was fascinated to learn that trees can communicate with each other, and that they support one another as a group along with other structures in the forest to ensure their survival. I was interested in the structure of the trees and how they were able to place themselves at equal distances from each other. I was also aware of the invasive species in the area that I walked in, and I noticed how their growing patterns were slightly different. It is amazing to understand that the forest functions as a true supportive community, including both plants and animals, and even though I have now walked this same trail hundreds of times, there are no two days that are exactly the same, and my personal reaction to the environment varies from day to day depending on what I encounter.

Based on this research, I wrote an article for the *Huffington Post* entitled "Using Exercise to Enhance Your Brain Power." This was in 2011, and I was becoming very frustrated by the growing obesity crisis across North America, especially amongst children. The public school systems across Canada had been threatening to limit students' physical activity opportunities (again) along with decreasing their time for free play outside. Movement, free play and unstructured learning opportunities offer ideal environments for education and brain development, but these ideas are often halted through politics and bureaucratic logistics. In the article I suggested that the two hours of physical activity per week required by most schools is not nearly adequate. I also suggested that everyone should spend more time in nature. To this day, I have yet to find or experience any research or observations that would suggest otherwise.

Early Years in Toronto

As I mentioned in a previous chapter, my first few years living in Toronto were filled with an excess amount of stress that was not healthy. I was hospitalized three times with chronic strep infections that could only be treated through IV antibiotics. I was teaching as a sessional lecturer at the University of Toronto and was missing way too many classes and deadlines as a result of these hospitalizations; that sad fact simply added to my overall stress. My husband and I had been separated for approximately six months, and although we were

Good relationships are
key to a healthy life,
but I also believe effective
stress management
and adequate amounts
of time spent outdoors
are essential.

———————

still talking on the phone, we were living alone in a big city where we knew very few people. I knew I had to make some big changes if I was going to continue living in this city.

I called a friend who was an ear, nose and throat (ENT) specialist in Saskatoon and asked him to refer me to a good ENT in Toronto. It turned out that his brother-in-law was a practising ENT at North York General Hospital, and thankfully, he was willing to see me on short notice. After taking one look at my tonsils and hearing my lengthy medical history, he booked me for surgery to have them removed within the next couple of weeks. I was relieved to be taking a step in a positive direction and hopefully toward improving my overall health.

Tim drove me home from the hospital following my surgery, and at this vulnerable time I just did not have it in me to argue about anything or even discuss the current state of our relationship. We had been living apart for many months prior to this surgery. I was happy to see him and extremely grateful that he was willing to help me get past this exhausting situation. We still did not completely understand what we needed to do to repair our broken relationship, but at this point we were both willing to work on whatever it took to improve our stressful lifestyle. Over the next few months, we made a much larger effort to change our habits and find ways to spend more time relaxing and enjoying each other's company instead of just working. As weeks together turned into months, we both found that these changes and insights improved our health, resilience and overall well-being.

The most obvious change we made in our lives at that time was that we went from a period where we spent basically no time in nature and shifted to a daily routine that involved way more outdoor time. The results were impressive. I decided that I would walk home from work instead of driving or taking transit, and on most days this took over an hour. I was also training a few clients for marathons at this time. I certainly did not need to add the extra mileage, but the mental health benefits were worth it. During my many lengthy walks home from work, I could feel my head clear in the fresh evening air; I loved walking through the various neighbourhoods of Toronto, and I enjoyed watching the gardens and flowers change as spring approached. These long walks allowed me to walk through the door to our home having already processed any stress related to my day at work or whatever else happened to be on my mind at the time. I would arrive home completely famished, enjoy having dinner and catching up with Tim and then basically collapse into a very contented, deep sleep.

Tim and I were slowly building a community of good friends in Toronto, and on a few occasions we were invited to cottages or farms for the weekend. We began to familiariże ourselves with the stunning landscapes north of Toronto, and we also realized how much we needed these breaks away from the noise and traffic of the city. We could almost feel our tension lifting as we drove to the outskirts of the city and found a quiet open road ahead of us. This time alone in the car also allowed us to communicate better and start to rebuild our relationship. I am incredibly grateful that we were able to find our way back to nature and eventually back to each other before it was too late.

Based on the unexpected results of the Harvard men's study—that one of the most important predictors of overall health is the quality of our relationships—and because most of us have probably spent some time in a toxic relationship, it is easy to understand how bad relationship stress can be for both your emotional and physical health. However, based on my personal experience, I do believe that a good relationship may not be the whole story. Those first couple of years living in Toronto, Tim and I had a great relationship, but at the same time we were both suffering from major issues of stress management that almost completely derailed our marriage. Good relationships are key to a healthy life, but I also believe effective stress management and adequate amounts of time spent outdoors are essential.

Through the wonders of social media (perhaps proving that it is not *always* bad), a close friend recently tagged me on a beautiful story she had posted about walking in a forest. This friend was going through a stressful divorce at the time, and although her career and family demanded most of her time, she occasionally was able to accompany me on my walks through the ravine, on weekends or over the holidays. She understood my devotion to nature and how I guarded this precious time in my daily routine. As I read the essay she sent, I found myself nodding at the beautiful words written by its insightful author. I have included part of this inspiring essay below, but I encourage you to read it in full whenever you have the chance. The author is Harry J. Stead, a writer from West Yorkshire, England.

> As far as I can tell, each of us seems to have a primal drive toward life, which finds its easiest expression in the act of walking, in the act of moving forward through the natural world and marvelling at its beauty. In my experience, all anxious and depressive feelings seem to dissipate when walking along a woodland path. And if you walk far enough you eventually achieve a state of joy—a quiet, inner happiness—and you are relieved, as you have escaped the walls, the squares, the eternity of sitting, of stagnation; now you are moving over the landscape, over the hills and far away, fighting against gravity, breathing fresh air, with a pulsing heart and an appetite for flowers and sunlight. You are free in search of the springs of life. A long walk is a rebirth of consciousness; one never returns quite the same, and is always better off for it.

This paragraph captures exactly how I feel after my daily walks in nature. As I read this article for the first time, my instinctual drive for connection also made me joyful to think that other human beings might experience similar feelings as they walk through forests or other natural landscapes. In our current technology-driven society, I am finding more support from all types of insightful people all over the world, including scientists, celebrities, artists, therapists and many others, who believe we need to spend more time in nature to improve our health, performance and happiness.

A wonderful summary of these ideas can be found in a recent book by Florence Williams entitled *The Nature Fix: Why Nature Makes Us Happier, Healthier, and More Creative*. Williams is a professional journalist who writes for several publications, including *National Geographic* and *Outside* magazine. What I love about her story is that she starts in a similar situation to the one Tim and I found ourselves in, moving to Toronto and abandoning our rural and outdoor roots. Williams had spent many years in Colorado, with a stunning backdrop of mountains close to her home. Because of a work opportunity for her husband, she finds herself living in Washington, DC. She then sets out on an epic journey around the world to find out why living in this noisy city is making her feel so awful. From forest bathing in Japan to the Cypress Forests of Korea and even a trip to Scotland to understand how they use nature to enhance treatment of mental illness, Williams has unearthed the science and data that help explain the positive effects we experience when we spend time in nature. Some of these benefits include improvements in our hormonal profile, decreases in our blood pressure and even the absorption from trees of aerosols that enhance our immunity.

A fascinating section of the book talks about how important nature is for children, and Williams explores how some countries are using time spent in nature to treat ADHD and depression in younger populations. The incidence of ADHD and depression have been steadily growing over the past decades. According to statistics from the US Centers for Disease Control and Prevention (CDC), 4.4 million children between the ages of 2 and 17 were diagnosed with ADHD in 2003, and by 2011 this number had grown to 6.4 million. Boys are significantly more likely than girls to be diagnosed with ADHD. Along with these troubling statistics, I am sure the rising levels of obesity in our younger populations in North America are a related trend. I cannot think of a more urgent and formative time of a person's life than childhood, when we are constantly testing and adapting our instinctual patterns. Our fast-paced, highly programmed, technology-driven atmosphere has been proven many times over to not be the most effective way to improve the health of the next generation. It is frustrating to think how many similar studies or population statistics it will take before we start to make significant changes that will be able to reverse these negative trends.

If we accept that nature and time spent outdoors are beneficial for both our mental and physical well-being, and if we were to compare the lives of our ancestors even 100 years ago with the amount of time most of us spend outdoors today, I am confident we would find a dramatic and troubling shift in our behaviours. Based on the current science, this shift away from nature will cause an increase in our negative stress hormones, a decrease in our overall immunity and a decrease in our capacity for creative thinking. You could also reasonably argue that if you are spending more time indoors, you may not be as active on a daily basis as you would be if you were outside more often. However, I am also aware of the challenges these ideas can present for most of our human population. Many of our common outdoor leisure activities are only available to members of the population who can afford both the time and the equipment. Things like downhill skiing, golf, fishing and even hunting come to mind. Adventure travel and eco travel are the fastest-growing segments of tourism, but again you must be able to afford both the time off work and the trip. A lifestyle that includes both the time and the financial means for these pursuits is generally available to only an exceedingly small percentage of our societies.

The good news is that to experience the positive health benefits from time spent in nature, you do not need to go to these extreme levels of immersion. Several research studies have indicated that we will see positive chemical and physiological changes in our body after only 20 minutes in nature. If you live in a larger city, you may need to become a bit more strategic about where you get your daily dose of "vitamin N," but this instinctual need represents a clear case where "the science has spoken," and you will only gain by listening to the results.

TRAINING TOOL: Spending More Time in Nature

My daily walk in the ravine is basically free. I schedule it around my work hours, so my only payment is sometimes a bit less sleep if I am starting my hike before an early workday. One of the studies presented in Williams's book suggests that positive health benefits can be found after only five more hours per month spent in nature. I feel this should be manageable for almost everyone, and because we know these effects may be even more important for children, time in nature should become a priority for everyone in your family; hopefully, this shift in thinking will make it easier for everyone to find the time. However, if finding time is the major obstacle when it comes to your immersion in nature, plan your breaks, weekends and maybe even some vacations with a focus on nature. As a result of the COVID-19 pandemic, we are currently limited by government travel restrictions. There is no better time to explore your own country! We have seen RV sales skyrocket and campgrounds reach capacity as a result. I am hoping this trend will continue and we will soon find ourselves with a whole new generation of outdoor enthusiasts.

RECOMMENDED READING: *The Nature Fix: Why Nature Makes Us Happier, Healthier, and More Creative* by Florence Williams

12

—

Instincts for Recovery and Rest

*The diseases which destroy
a man are no less natural than the
instincts which preserve him.*

GEORGE SANTAYANA,
DIALOGUES IN LIMBO

OFTEN, WHEN YOU are living through a stressful time in your life, you are too involved with the current situation to be able to sense how your body is reacting to it in a physiological way. As is often the case, when you are busy trying to survive a pandemic, impress a new boss or simply fit in, that becomes your primary focus, and other aspects of your life can suffer.

A certain level of stress is essential for all human survival. However, we were designed to survive our stress and then rest and recover so as to be ready for the next stressful situation. This is exactly the method we use when we are working with elite athletes. You apply various stressors to their movement systems and sometimes even cognitive stresses related to the demands of their sport, and then you structure the best possible environment for them to rest and recover. When they return, their body has improved through the remarkable process of adaptation. Optimal recovery time can be applied to almost all areas of our lives. Anyone who has sat through a two- or even three-hour meeting can attest to the fact that this is too long for us to be able to pay proper attention to something. Instead, most businesses and academic institutions know that 50 minutes is a reasonable amount of time for humans to work or concentrate, followed by a 10-minute break or rest, after which you will be ready for a better performance in the next 50 minutes. Without a proper recovery, the second or third hour of a meeting is possibly wasted because efficiency and effectiveness are drastically diminished.

If the rest and recovery period of any type of training, whether it is physical or mental, is inadequate before the next stress is encountered, you will eventually see a breakdown instead of an adaptation. The greatest advances in sports science related to training athletes at the Olympic and professional levels have focused on improvements in the effectiveness of recovery. Many professional sports scandals have revealed the dedicated science behind illegal methods used to improve athletic performance by means of pharmaceutical interventions. In many cases these substances are not taken during competitions, because they do not usually affect the athlete's competition performance, but rather are designed to be used as part of the pre-competition training, with the goal of drastically improving the athlete's recovery and adaptation to high volumes of training.

As training techniques and strategies evolve, we see more extensive, and entirely legal, strategies filter down from high-performance athletics into the mainstream population. Much media attention has been devoted to the "groundbreaking" recovery techniques practised by one of the world's most phenomenal basketball players, LeBron James. Many scientists and coaches working in sports science research will agree that his results are powerful every time he steps on the court. According to these sources, James spends over seven figures per year on his overall body care. He has been quoted emphasizing that sleep is more important than many of the latest and greatest techniques he employs. Here is a small glimpse into some of the recovery strategies used by James as he talks about the importance of a good night's sleep:

That's the best way for your body to physically and emotionally be able to recover and get back to 100 percent as possible. Now, will you wake up and feel 100 percent? There are some days you don't. So some days you feel better than others. But the more, and more, and more time that you get those eight—if you can get nine, that's amazing... I could do all the ice bags and the NormaTecs and everything that we do, that we have as far as our recovery package, while I'm up... But when you get in that good sleep, you just wake up, and you feel fresh. You don't need an alarm clock. You just feel like, "Okay. I can tackle this day at the highest level."

In general, human beings will thrive in an environment where we are recovering well from whatever stressors we are encountering on a regular basis. Our instincts for rest and recovery are incredibly important to our overall health and performance. I believe this is one area where we have managed to seriously damage our health in Western society.

Although sleep and recovery are essential, they are not the complete picture. We all know people who often get more than the required amounts of sleep and rest but who are not always the picture of health and productivity.

If we are looking at recovery as a strategy for performance and health, we need to understand that not all methods are created equal. Sleep is recorded in several stages, most commonly four or five (depending on what research you are looking at). During a typical night where you have eight hours of sleep, you should cycle through these stages approximately four to six times. Each stage affects different parts of our body and brain, and it seems that all the stages are essential for effective rest. While we sleep, our body repairs physical damage done to cells, our brain sorts and even "prunes" our thoughts and visual inputs from the day, and our neuromuscular system replenishes its nutrients to be ready for the next time it is needed. Those are just a few of the many physiological functions that occur while we are sleeping; there are many more, depending on the needs of your body on a particular night.

Our instincts for rest
and recovery are incredibly
important to our overall
health and performance.

———————

I am sure you have experienced how good you feel when you wake up from a fantastic night of rest, and how tired you feel after a horrible one. There is a reason sleep deprivation is used as a form of torture: lack of sleep can be extremely damaging to us on many levels. Anyone who has cared for a newborn, a puppy or aging parents will have experienced how exhausting it can be when you are required to wake up many times through the night; sometimes you feel more tired in the morning than you did the previous night. People who travel to different time zones on a regular basis often face extreme challenges from the constant disruption to their sleeping patterns and circadian rhythms. Sleep apnea, alcohol consumption, an uncomfortable temperature, emotional stress, chronic pain or even loud city noise can prevent many sleepers from reaching the deep cycles we need to recover properly from the everyday demands of life. The negative health impacts of shift work have been well documented over the last few decades. One of the first homes we lived in when we moved to Toronto was very close to an active train track. To drown out the noise from the trains, we ran our window air conditioner all night every night—even in the winter. Both Tim and I realized after we moved to a quieter neighbourhood that the trains barrelling through our old neighbourhood had been waking us up a couple of times a night. After a few nights in our new location, we both realized we were waking up more rested.

The CDC has listed airline attendants' work schedules as a risk factor because of significant increases in various types of cancer. As part of the research explanation, it says that this risk is possibly a result of the regular disruption of the workers' circadian rhythms. Research continues in this area, as scientists try to understand the causal relationship between sleep disruption and increased incidence of various cancers.

It is likely that we will all live through periods of our lives where we are not able to get enough quality sleep, rest or recovery. We have created a 24-hour society where we can shop, gamble and even do a workout at any hour of the day or night. As a result, the health of our populations is suffering. The most important thing you can do regarding your rest and recovery is form a strategy. Make sure you are not chronically sleep deprived. Learn how to meditate or take a catnap so you can use these techniques on days when your sleep was less than optimal. Relying on stimulants such as caffeine or other pharmaceuticals is not an effective way to manage sleep deprivation. If you prioritize your sleep and practise good sleep hygiene, you will soon notice the numerous benefits. Maybe one day we can hope for results as awesome as LeBron James's!

TRAINING TOOL: Recovery and Rest

Recognizing the importance of recovery is essential for optimal performance in every aspect of our lives. Lack of sleep is linked to depression, cancer, obesity, cardiovascular disease and many other significant health problems. In North America we are currently described as a "sleep-deprived" society. Once you understand that sleep and rest are essential, you must then find a way to incorporate them into your daily rituals, which are hopefully structured in a way that honours your basic instincts. All adults require 7 to 8 hours of restful sleep per night, and children require 10 to 11 (when they are growing). If we do not meet these requirements, things begin to break down. It is as simple as that. There are several great resources on this topic that have obsessed scientists for centuries. If you are lacking sleep, please prioritize a positive change in this area above all the other instincts we are talking about. It is that important.

If you are going through a period where a good night's sleep is not an option, for example shift work or caring for a newborn, try to develop techniques such as meditation or restful breaks that you can add to your daily recovery time. If the changes to your sleep patterns are temporary, you will be able to use these techniques to help you perform to the best of your ability until the situation improves.

RECOMMENDED READING: *The Sleep Revolution: Transforming Your Life, One Night at a Time* by Arianna Huffington

13
—

Instincts and Physical Performance

Human beings are born with the instinct to express themselves through movement. Even before he could communicate with words, primitive man was dancing to the beat of his own heart.

BOB FOSSE

WHY IS MOVEMENT so critical to our health and well-being? Many scientists, doctors and fitness enthusiasts have pondered this question in all sorts of ways for decades. The one thing that inevitably comes up in any discussion of our overall health, and which all agree is a major positive influencer of "wellness," is regular movement. And yet, as each year passes, we seem to move less.

Humans have evolved from walking up to roughly 16 kilometres (10 miles) a day during our time as hunters and gatherers to less than 3 kilometres (2 miles) per day (on average) in our current lifestyle. We have been overcome by a wave of sedentary work environments and entertainment habits. It is difficult to imagine or understand the massive health implications resulting from this incredible change, which has taken place over a relatively short time period when you consider our evolution as a species.

At a very basic level, the human body was designed to be in constant slow, repetitive movement during the day, followed by sleep for eight to ten hours at night to allow for full recovery and repair and to be ready for the same demands the next day. Occasionally our bodies would need to supply rapid bursts of energy when there was a greater demand for speed or strength, and there were also periods of sitting and resting as we ate or simply relaxed. Our lifestyle today does not

169

remotely resemble what we were designed for or are capable of based on the historical challenges of daily life.

Possibly the best way to understand how this affects our physical and mental health is to find people who currently live a lifestyle that does require very regular movement and then compare this population with our inactive majority. These highly active populations do exist, in our marathon runners and endurance athletes, and even within careers that require constant motion as a part of the daily job requirement.

A large-scale study in Finland evaluated 2,613 elite male athletes divided into three different groups depending on their sport history (power athletes, team sport athletes and endurance athletes). The endurance athletes competed in sports such as marathons, long-distance running and cross-country skiing—sub-maximal exercise or training that lasts for long periods of time throughout the day.

The researchers then compared the lifespan of these elite athletes with that of 1,712 ordinary Finnish men who were not competitive athletes. The findings were as follows:

- Power athletes lived 1.6 years longer
- Team athletes lived 4 years longer
- Endurance athletes lived 5.7 years longer

Finding a way to potentially increase your lifespan by six years is something almost everyone should be interested in. However, despite the fact that the evidence supporting the health benefits of regular daily exercise is overwhelming, many humans choose not to participate. This challenging behaviour trait is something that defies logic and again points to a need to gain a better understanding of how our instincts are related to our movement behaviours (or lack of such).

A large-scale study utilizing data from mobile devices studied a data set consisting of 68 million days of physical activity for 717,527 people, providing a window into activity in 111 countries across the globe. A goal of the study was to increase awareness and understanding of global rates of inactivity, which, the researchers suggest, currently leads to an additional 53 million deaths per year. The highest-scoring country in this study was Japan, with an average of 6,000 steps per day, while the lowest activity score was recorded by Saudi Arabia, with an average of 3,500 steps per day. North Americans scored somewhere in the middle, at around 4,500 to 5,000 steps per day (which translates into less than 4 kilometres (2.5 miles) of walking per day). As we would suspect, the countries with lower activity had higher levels of obesity, cancer and cardiovascular disease.

Another valuable piece of data provided by this study found that participants living in the most "walkable" cities in the world did have higher levels of activity. San Francisco, California, has been voted one of the most walkable cities on the planet, and the activity levels recorded in that city were some of the highest in the study.

As we search for strategies to improve our instinctual movement behaviours, it is important to find the factors that have an actual positive impact. Solutions can be as simple as living in an environment that supports and promotes walking, because we know this will increase your overall amount of daily activity. It is also important to emphasize that the simplest daily movements have a beneficial impact on our overall health. This differs from our previous belief that in order to be healthy, we had to engage in things that were considered "workouts" or "exercise." We now know there are benefits to simply being more active every day.

A recent study published in the *Journal of the American College of Cardiology* evaluated 138 novice runners as they trained to complete a marathon (42 kilometres/26.2 miles). Marathon training drastically increases your overall movement during the day, and as the volume increases, we could argue that although you are not moving as much as we may have done in prehistoric times, you are definitely adding to your daily mileage in a very significant way. These researchers focused their investigation on the impact of this training on the participants' heart health, and they found that on average the runners were able to reverse the aging process in their heart by approximately four years. A part of the study that I found particularly interesting indicated that the most significant benefit was found in the group of men who were slower runners, indicating that slower methodical movements are possibly more beneficial to our overall health.

Our company, Totum Life Science, employs some of the best practitioners of movement science, rehabilitation, coaching and personal training in the country. Every day, we are presented with the challenge of overcoming barriers to regular movement. The barrier could be owing to a fracture from a fall, an injury related to chronic overtraining, or sometimes simply problems with motivation or confidence that decrease someone's ability to move regularly. While we may employ the latest technology in imaging, fancy gadgets and amazing treatment protocols, our main goal is simply to keep people moving as best we can. We know from both experience and science that this is what matters most to a patient's physical and mental well-being.

Our basic human movement patterns are amazing capabilities we are all born with. They are critically important to our longevity and quality of life. One of the most common statements I make to my patients and training clients is: *Momentum is everything.*

The reason I repeat this line is that, as I have experienced during my times off with various injuries, and as you may have experienced yourself at various challenging times in your life, it is so much easier to maintain movement proficiency than to build it again once it has been lost. Maintaining good health is infinitely easier than working your way back to a healthy lifestyle and avoiding old temptations. Maintaining a healthy body weight is so much easier than losing excess weight. You get the picture.

When it comes to human movement, I am a huge fan of the basics. These things are not sexy and they will not get you tons of new followers if you decide to post them on Instagram. However, I am sure you will agree that being able to run, squat, walk and jump will always be

Momentum
is everything.

---

more useful to you in regular life than having the ability to perform "10 Variations of the Most Perfect Butt-Blasting Lifts."

Hundreds of years ago, movements were trained by enhancing basic movement patterns using extraordinarily little equipment or technology. Sports were invented with a focus on who was the best at these simple movements, and games evolved out of leisurely or friendly competitions. Fighting, wrestling, boxing and jousting were a big part of athletic contests during this time, and even man versus beast was a part of the brutal Roman gladiator spectacles. Training for these various contests was partially incorporated into everyday physical labour. Men who lifted very heavy things as a part of their daily routine would be champions at feats of strength. Men whose daily activity involved miles of running would be good at the endurance events, while men who were regularly called upon as the warriors of the tribe or community, or later as soldiers in fist-to-fist combat, became very proficient at the combative competitions.

Sports as entertainment remained in this basic arena for hundreds of years, eventually becoming highly organized as populations found value and enjoyment in these types of events, as both spectators and participants. The ancient Olympic Games began as early as 776 BC in Olympia, Greece. The first modern Olympic Games took place in Athens, Greece, in 1896. Soon the champions of these various events became heroes to their communities, and everyone wanted to look like these muscular athletes who were dominating these spectacles of human movement and performance.

Late in the 19th century we see the first examples of public performances that were designed simply to show the audience what a perfect male physique is supposed to look like. The first documented athlete in this sphere was Eugen Sandow, who promoted his "perfect" physique on various stages throughout England. Sandow and his performances became so popular that he was able to develop a full training system, including dumbbells and pulleys, that was sold to the masses. His body was defined as the perfect "Grecian" physique, around which measurements and standards were formed to identify what the ideal male should look like.

Even though the training programs designed by Sandow were based on the attainment of a very specific physical look or aesthetic, we can still see the huge influence of this type of bodybuilding training all over the world. Today, most gyms and fitness facilities still have equipment designed to enhance your muscles through body-building exercises, along with a few pieces designed for powerlifting, such as the bench press and squats. It is important to understand that many of these fancy machines are designed to train a specific muscle or group of muscles in isolation. To this day, you can walk into any large gym facility and find a group of people (mostly guys) who have exceptionally large, muscular upper bodies and much smaller and less impressive lower bodies. We can all see that this style of isolation training is very effective for making people look different, but in many cases it is very ineffective for human performance if we think back to our basic movement patterns and our ability to function well in our own environments.

Although training the basics may not look fancy, and it is certainly not headline-grabbing in our current climate, where we can find a new trendy training technique for every day of the week, in my experience it is essential and efficient. Part of the reason for its efficiency is that we already have these movement patterns in our brain; the training is designed to refine and improve them. This style of training is also the *most* effective because these are the movements your anatomy is already designed to perform, and these are the movements you should be performing daily. It is super-important that you have a deep understanding of them, and hopefully with a bit of extra effort and practice you will be able to perform them with great proficiency throughout your *whole* life.

Basic Instinctual Movement Patterns

Human beings are born with approximately 19 movement patterns:

1 Crawling
2 Walking
3 Running
4 Climbing
5 Squatting
6 Jumping
7 Pushing
8 Pulling
9 Throwing
10 Catching
11 Lifting something overhead
12 Reaching to grab something (this could include things on the ground or overhead)
13 Striking
14 Digging
15 Rotating through the torso to gain momentum to throw or hit something (twisting)
16 Dancing
17 Swimming
18 Skating
19 Skiing

When we are children, we can usually execute most of these basic movements with adequate proficiency even though we have never been taught or coached how to do them. We probably do not know why we should try to be good at these things, and we often take them for granted, as they are just part of being human.

Human movement provides an excellent opportunity to understand and study the potential of human instincts when we work to enhance them as much as we possibly can. For example, most of us have the basic pattern to run. If we then look at a group of world-class sprinters, we see that their running resembles something completely different from the original movement pattern that many of us use when we try to run. The sprinters have taken this basic movement pattern and practised it for hours upon hours, and days upon days. With every practice, the pattern improves. The connections in the sprinter's brain become stronger and they process these signals much faster than their fellow humans. They have taken the basic instinct for running and turned it into a "superpower" through repetitive practice, dedicated learning and hard work.

If we then look at a group of marathon runners, we find a similar pattern. They took the movement pattern for running that was in their body and brain. They then began to test how long they could keep running before they had to stop from exhaustion. Slowly, their brain adapted their pathway to make them very efficient at running long distances. With repetition, their brain also helped develop other aspects of their body to accommodate the demands of running long distances. They turned their instinctual ability for running into an amazing talent for endurance.

We can look at every movement pattern and find similar examples of awesomeness achieved through training and repetition: MLB pitchers for throwing, NFL players for catching, NBA players for reaching to grab something, Olympic weightlifters for pushing, and the list goes on. These exceptional human beings were born to the species *Homo sapiens* just like you and me. The big difference is that they develop an inherent drive to become extremely proficient at one of these instinctual movement patterns, or possibly a few of them. Then the question becomes one of nature versus nurture: what aspects of these athletes' environment contributed to their ability to excel at these particular movement patterns, and what motivated them to groove these patterns into their brains and bodies to this level? In movement and athletics, we will find many examples to support the theory that our environment plays a much larger part in our long-term success than our genetics.

When I think of an environment that encouraged great athletic performances, the Williams sisters immediately spring to mind. Like most of us, I had a childhood that was drastically different from the environment Serena and Venus Williams grew up in, and it is easy to understand why they are unstoppable forces on the tennis court while I struggle to return a soft serve. When we look at movement proficiency and excellence, we can find many examples similar to these. The children of athletes tend to have more success in athletics all the way to the professional level. There is a disproportionately large number of children who make it to the NHL who are related to NHL players. Also, a disproportionate number of siblings play the same sport at the highest level. Most sports scientists will agree that although these athletes may have a slight genetic advantage, their exceptional results are more dependent on their environment and the time spent training as they grew up.

You may be thinking that you have absolutely no desire to train your movement instincts to the levels cited above. However, the important point to take away from these case studies is that movement patterns have the ability to be enhanced throughout most people's lifespan. Instead of having your fitness routine continually diverted by the latest gimmick, gadget or fad, shift your focus to perfecting your basic movement patterns first. There are innumerable ways for you to move your body and exercise. By mastering the basics first, you will be able to expand your repertoire to include movements you would like to do for fun, while at the same time lowering your risk of being injured when you dive into a new sport. On a very practical level, it would be helpful to have someone watch you perform all of these basic movement patterns and then help you discover what areas need to be improved to enhance your overall health.

At our company, we have a protocol called a functional movement screen, and I am confident that many places around the world also offer this service. The functional movement screen is a good place to start to examine some of your basic movement patterns, understand where you have challenges and then develop ways to improve. Another great source of information for many of us is a gait analysis carried out by an experienced professional. Most of us will need to walk and occasionally run throughout our lifetime, so it is an excellent idea to spend some time becoming more efficient at this.

If we agree with the theory that exceptional performance in sports, the arts and possibly even business is acquired through practice, repetition and hard work, we can then put together a plan to improve these instinctual patterns in all areas of our life. Again, it is a matter of understanding how to harness and emphasize the superpowers that are already inside you.

Instincts for Efficiency

There exists one major caveat to the idea that we will be healthier if we move more. Our ancient ancestors were forced to move for most of the day because this was how they were able to get food and water and basically survive the environment they lived in. At the same time, our bodies are designed to conserve energy when we have the opportunity. Getting adequate rest would have been an especially important survival strategy thousands of years ago. If you could only find so much food or water for any particular day, it would be ridiculous to waste your energy and calories running around for no particular reason; instead, you were designed to rest when it was safe to rest and move when you needed to. This urge to conserve energy is still a dominant part of our daily movement patterns.

When most of us step onto a bus or subway, we scan the area for a place to sit down. When we must walk from one location to another, our brain immediately tries to figure out the shortest route possible. There is a whole area of industrial design focused on finding ways to make our daily habits and movements more efficient. We now have robots and appliances that will handle many daily chores that would require extra movement from us during our day, and the more efficient these inventions are, the greater the market for them becomes.

Today it is hard to imagine getting up to change a channel on your television or leaving the couch to answer your phone, but these movements were part of our daily routines 30 or 40 years ago. It is possible that my house would go into complete lockdown amid formal protests if I asked my children to wash all our dishes by hand.

It is crucial to our overall health and performance that we figure out ways to enjoy ourselves while regularly repeating our basic movement patterns.

———————

I am exposed to variations of this energy-conserving instinct every day at work. Often, when I prescribe a certain exercise, I am looking at strengthening a specific part of someone's body either to improve their performance or to help them recover from an injury. Almost without fail, the learning pattern will go as follows:

1   I will demonstrate the exercise and explain what area we are trying to train so as to improve a patient's movement pattern.

2   I will have the patient show me the same exercise to see that they understand what I am explaining to them.

3   Most of the time, these exercises must be repeated, and I will ask the patient to keep doing the exercise until I ask them to stop.

4   The first five repetitions will look like what I have demonstrated. Then, in most cases, I will see the movement change because my patient has figured out a way to do it more easily. In typical gym talk, we call this "cheating" an exercise.

5   Once this cheating starts, I will ask the patient to stop. We will review the exercise, talk about what part they were not doing correctly and try again. Depending on the patient and their attention to detail, this process can repeat itself many times before they eventually perform the exercise the correct way.

The reason this takes so long is that I am forcing them to go against their instinct to be efficient. In fact, with many training exercises I am looking for a non-efficient way to move, because I am trying to fix a problematic movement pattern, and in order to do this, we must work hard to groove a new neural movement pathway.

This example highlights one of the major challenges we face as a society when we talk about ways to improve our overall health. Most people are more inclined to rest than to move. In fact, of the people I work with and the patients I see (excluding professional athletes, or fitness instructors who are paid to move), the only ones who actually make a point of moving every day are the people who have discovered and fully believe in the lifestyle benefits movement brings.

"Movement Is Medicine" is a quote I often see in social media posts, or in magazines promoting fitness or health habits. Over the last 100 years, science has demonstrated that by participating in regular daily movement along with an occasional bout of more intense exercise, we will enjoy numerous benefits to our health, performance and even happiness. There are many examples from real life that demonstrate "movement" as one of the most powerful medicines you could ever take. The problem with this concept is that we are used to taking most types of medicine in the form of a pill, which produces results immediately (or promises to); with exercise, the rewards are less obvious, and may be drawn out over a lifetime. Our fast-paced lifestyle, filled with devices that trigger immediate gratification, have trained us to crave a "quick fix" of serotonin or dopamine. Exercise will improve your hormonal profile in a similar way, but it takes at least 10 to 20 minutes before you feel it. Most of us simply do not want to wait that long.

There also exist some rare humans who are completely addicted to the adrenalin and mental shifts that exercise provides. These are the patients I regularly treat, who will run themselves into the ground before they give up that feeling of a "runner's high" or the full-body relaxation that a good workout provides. Exercise can become an addiction in some isolated cases. As with any type of addiction, we can identify this problem when we see that a person is exercising in a way that is detrimental to their overall health and is also interfering with other positive aspects of their life.

This phenomenon is quite different from the "overtraining" we commonly see with competitive athletes. In most cases a good coach will have various techniques and tests to identify a situation of overtraining. One simple technique is to take a regular measurement of heart rate variability. With the fast-developing world of wearable technology, we will soon be able to determine the exact dose of each type of exercise that is ideal for our unique genetic code.

Devices can now inform us about how much we are moving each day, how many calories we are burning and whether or not we are getting good-quality sleep. I have tested many of these devices and I do find that they are fun to use for a while, but I believe it is more important to understand what your body feels like when you are in a good pattern of exercise and rest. This feeling does come back to our ability to listen to our instincts to move and to rest. Once we can do this, we will not need to rely on devices to constantly track us, because we will know instinctively what is best.

TRAINING TOOL: Instincts for Physical Performance

Exercise and movement are powerful healers of the human body, and our bodies were designed to be in regular movement for as much of the day as possible. It is crucial to our overall health and performance that we figure out ways to enjoy ourselves while regularly repeating our basic movement patterns. Once we understand that we are born with several basic movement patterns, it becomes a completely worthwhile endeavour to do our best to enhance or improve these patterns. For example, what if over the next six months you dedicated some time to improving your running technique? You may not become a world-class sprinter, but you could possibly improve your speed and efficiency by about 30 percent. That running skill then becomes a practical tool that can last you a lifetime.

When we participate in games or activities that we love, exercise and movement also have the ability to enhance our happiness and add to our feelings of connection. If you have ever won some type of physical competition as part of a team, you will understand what I am talking about. This does not mean that you must strive to compete at the highest levels; in fact, some of our elite athletes find that they lose the enjoyment of their sport amidst the politics, stress and money involved at the top levels. To get a feeling of the true joy of exercise, watch a group of teenagers competing in a playground basketball pickup game, or if you live through a freezing cold winter as I do, take yourself to an outdoor rink to watch a neighbourhood game of shinny. If you take the time to carefully and quietly watch, you will hopefully see and feel a poetic quality of movement on display that comes from an instinctual human desire to play, move and connect with each other. Movement and performance can be as simple and as beautiful as that.

RECOMMENDED READING: *Movement: Functional Movement Systems: Screening, Assessment, and Corrective Strategies* by Gray Cook; *Becoming a Supple Leopard: The Ultimate Guide to Resolving Pain, Preventing Injury, and Optimizing Athletic Performance* by Kelly Starrett with Glen Cordoza

14

Instinctual Eating

Let food be thy medicine
and medicine be thy food.

HIPPOCRATES

GOOD NUTRITION IS an essential part of every human being's existence. When we are eating well, we tend to thrive in our daily lives, but when we are regularly lacking important nutrients, we are more likely to become ill and, eventually, die. For most humans, eating consumes a large portion of each day. We make regular decisions about where we are going to eat, what we will eat, where to get our food, how to prepare it and whom we will eat it with. Eating is an instinctual behaviour that begins the minute we are born. Many new parents are shocked at how highly motivated a newborn baby can be with respect to its nourishment. If you manage to screw up any part of the feeding (as I did regularly as a new mom), you will be faced with an extremely angry, red-faced, screaming baby. When you get it right, you are rewarded with a blissful, sleepy baby.

During our first year of life, we spend most of our time eating and sleeping. Eating behaviours are remarkably simple to begin with, but this instinctual pattern becomes much more complicated as we age—especially in our modern civilized culture. The way we eat today is vastly different from the habits and structures around eating of our ancient ancestors, who foraged, hunted and consumed the food they found necessary for survival.

As we try to optimize our health, performance and happiness, we must include a strategy for nutrition, because it is essential to everything we do and because our energy levels depend on it. As discussed earlier, agricultural practices drastically altered the lives of human beings, in terms of how we found and consumed our food. It is also important to understand that the consumption of food represents a massive part of our economy, and so the motivation behind food production is vastly different today compared with hundreds of years ago.

The value of global food and agricultural production for 2018 totalled about $8.7 trillion, or about 10 percent of the world's GDP. As the earth's population continues to grow, it is quite probable that these numbers will also continue to increase. Food and agricultural exports are one of the biggest businesses in North America. As revenues continue to grow, the companies involved in this industry will continue to look for ways to improve their efficiencies, production levels and profits. Often, however, profits and quality, or nutritional value, are in direct opposition when we are talking about food production and agriculture. Mass production and distribution of food can compromise its nutritional value. Owing to the travel and factory-like conditions that characterize modern food production, ingredients such as antibiotics and preservatives have the potential to enter our diet in a significant way. Along with this come many extra ingredients that are added to our food to make it more palatable, and in some cases even addictive. Salt, sugar, fat and artificial colouring are some of the main ingredients scientifically manipulated in the processed food industry, with a goal of enticing us to eat more and hopefully buy more as we grow to love these tastes, colours and textures.

Michael Moss wrote an extremely enlightening book on this topic, *Salt, Sugar, Fat: How the Food Giants Hooked Us*. In this book, he provides an excellent overview of the current state of the food industry in North America. Personally, although I was not surprised by the information, I was a bit frightened to learn of the lengths to which these companies and scientists will go. As Moss writes,

> Inevitably, the manufacturers of processed food argue that
> they have allowed us to become the people we want to be, fast

and busy, no longer slaves to the stove. But in their hands, the salt, sugar, and fat they have used to propel this social transformation are not nutrients as much as weapons—weapons they deploy, certainly, to defeat their competitors but also to keep us coming back for more.

The main problem I see with our current style of eating is that it is not working for our overall health. Even though we are consuming way more calories each day, our blood work would indicate that many of us are missing out on key nutrients because of the lack of variety in our daily diet. I am sure this problem is based on two important variables. One is addiction. We are, for the most part, addicted to the taste of certain ingredients, such as sugar, fat and salt, to the point where, whenever we eat, our brain is telling us to find those tastes. The second variable is the way we take our food for granted. Most of us know that we are not at risk of starving, so we eat in a mindless manner in order to satisfy our feelings of hunger or boredom, without thinking too much about our nutritional intake. If we ever found ourselves in an environment where we believed we were at risk of starvation, I imagine our food intake practices would change drastically, moving quickly back to our patterns of instinctual eating. We would search out nutrient-rich foods and probably avoid overly processed foods because we would soon realize they did not provide us with enough nutrients to warrant them as a smart choice.

Moving back in time to a place where we felt unsure about where our next meal was coming from would be impractical and impossible, but we need to understand that our current system is not working. I am inspired by the many nutrition experts I work with regularly who demonstrate and teach our patients and clients better strategies for eating. There is a fast-growing part of our population that is working hard to produce locally grown and nutrient-dense food, and they are rewarded with customers willing to spend more money for better-quality food.

There is a fast-growing
part of our population that is
working hard to produce
locally grown and nutrient-
dense food, and they are
rewarded with customers
willing to spend more money
for better-quality food.

———————

When we are working with elite athletes at Totum, we often finish our training sessions with a plan for refuelling in the optimal way. This involves strategies for where we get our food and how we prepare it, and we even talk about the importance of taking the time to sit down (ideally with friends or family) to enjoy the food, as we bask in the knowledge that we are doing great things for our overall health and well-being.

When I do speaking engagements or lectures, I always try to save time at the end for questions. I love reflecting with the audience as we discuss various concepts related to health and exercise, and I always enjoy meeting new people and hearing different perspectives. Usually the first or second question will be about a new fad diet or something related to nutrition. Of course, this makes perfect sense: we are required to eat every single day, and most of us do it many times each day, so it should not be surprising that this topic takes up a big part of our brainpower!

My Personal (Extremely Sophisticated) Meal Plan

Prepare to be underwhelmed...

Morning

I do not usually eat breakfast, as I am busy in the morning getting my children fed and ready for school and getting myself ready for work. I am not very hungry in the morning either, so I prefer to eat later.

- 2 cups of coffee with milk, cream or almond milk
- 1 large glass of water with lemon, a powder that has green vegetables and cayenne pepper

Lunch

Usually leftovers from last night's dinner: could include tacos, chicken, potatoes, beans, pasta, salad, seafood casserole, chicken pot pie, fried fish, steak, hamburgers, chicken burgers, salmon burgers, Thai food, noodle-based dishes... Honestly, the list is very long, but also pretty basic.

I also usually have some type of dessert (cookie) or toast with peanut butter and honey.

Dinner

Similar to lunch. Always a protein with a couple of vegetables. We love all types of pasta; we eat many types of meat. We try to limit red meat to a couple of times per week and we try to have fish at least once a week. We will have a salad at dinner most nights and possibly some type of bread along with our meal. I do make a point of purchasing food locally as much as possible. We have good relationships with our butchers, our grocery store managers and a few farmers from whom we are able to purchase produce or meat directly. We care about the quality of our food and where it comes from, but nobody in our family is very picky and we all consume large quantities of food every day.

Dessert

Cookies, chocolate, banana bread, pie (strawberry rhubarb, my absolute favourite!) with ice cream, chocolate cake, carrot cake

Later evening snack

Chips, chocolate, nuts, cheese, grapes

During my conversations about food with athletes or in front of an audience, I am often asked how I eat. As you can see from the sidebar, I have a very basic eating style, with nothing too fancy or sophisticated about it. When we are entertaining, we do try to come up with things that are a bit more interesting, but this is our day-to-day, week-to-week eating style. My husband and I absolutely love all kinds of food, we love wine (and pretty much every type of cocktail), and we love entertaining. I think (hope) that our children have also learned these positive and rewarding feelings about food. We enjoy eating together as a family and we also enjoy exploring new restaurants or new types of food together.

The only challenging part of this way of eating relates to the decision we made once we had children that food, nutrition and eating together as a family would all be priorities in our lives. When you try your best to turn food into an enjoyable part of your day, it becomes something you look forward to instead of just a chore you must perform because you are hungry. Like most practices related to your health, once you make it a priority, you must then carve out the time in your busy schedule to make it happen. I will admit that, because of this, we are not the most productive human beings on the planet, but we are all enjoying our time spent eating and really doing simply fine with that.

Every day in my practice, with friends and sometimes even with colleagues who work in the fitness industry, I am reminded of how unhealthy our current human relationship with food can get. Our digitally driven, photo-sharing-obsessed society spends a significant amount of time evaluating photos of ourselves and others. It is hard to avoid a sense of being judged solely on what you look like. Working as an athlete and coach in track and field, figure skating and ballet, I was exposed to many athletes with disordered eating along with the often-associated diagnosis of body dysmorphic disorder (BDD), anorexia or bulimia. The saddest, most soul-crushing part of this to me is that because we have to eat many times a day, these disorders and obsessions have the ability to consume so much of a person's life.

At the other end of the spectrum, obesity is a growing problem in many first-world countries, with some of the most technologically advanced societies experiencing the worst levels. According to the World Health Organization, the prevalence of worldwide obesity tripled between 1975 and 2016. One of the most shocking revelations in this data from the WHO is that over 340 million children and adolescents aged 5 to 19 were overweight or obese in 2016. This fact makes me incredibly sad and frustrated about our current lifestyles as they relate to nutrition and activity, because in most of these cases the children do not have much control over what they eat and how much activity they get. They are simply caught up in a lifestyle that encourages sedentary behaviours along with inexpensive processed food.

How could instinctual eating change these severely negative health outcomes? For starters, obesity most likely did not exist in ancient times, because the effort involved in hunting and gathering food made it nearly impossible to become obese. I realize that we cannot turn the clock back to that way of life—nor would most people want to do that! We love the convenience of fast food; we also love the variety of food that is easily accessible whenever we want to eat. The massive food industry with its sophisticated marketing budgets encourages us to "never be hungry" and spreads the message that constant snacking is something we should all practise. These habits are almost impossible to break.

If we were going to set up the perfect environment for instinctual eating, it would probably look and feel like a highly active vacation. Our day might begin with a glass of water when we wake up, followed by a long hike through an ancient forest. Our light breakfast would include delicious protein and tons of hydration (we are normally dehydrated in the morning). This would be followed by approximately three hours of light activity: strolling through a museum, shopping in an outdoor market, productive things such as yard work or other chores that keep us moving, not sitting or sedentary. By lunchtime we would be hungry again, so we would take a break, ideally to eat garden-fresh vegetables, a protein and some type of fruit. Maybe we would rest after this meal or even have a short nap. The later afternoon would ideally involve some form of recreational activity; any type of competitive game we enjoyed would be perfect. At around 6 p.m.,

Instinctual eating
leads you to a healthy
relationship
with your food.

———————

we would begin to prepare a dinner with ingredients that we sourced locally. If this activity involved many members of our family or friends, that would be even better for our mental health. We would eat as many varieties of vegetable as possible, along with a high-quality protein and something sweet for dessert. Following the dinner cleanup (this counts as low-level movement) we would go for a leisurely stroll, and as it got dark, we would go to bed and fall into a deep sleep for eight to ten hours.

In a perfect world, this is what instinctual eating could look like. Unfortunately, very few of us live in a situation that resembles this. Maybe some of you have experienced this type of day while on vacation. Even though it is difficult to adhere to these concepts completely, we can break them down into smaller components that could be possible for most of us on some days:

- Go for a short walk before breakfast.

- Make sure your breakfast includes some healthy proteins.

- Source local and organic vegetables whenever possible.

- Try to eat as many varieties of vegetable as possible during the day.

- Keep moving as much as possible during the day.

- Make dinnertime a social event with either family or friends on as many days of the week as possible.

- Try to do some form of light activity at the end of your day: go for a walk, clean the kitchen or even organize a closet.

- Source local high-quality proteins (chicken, fish, pork or beef) whenever possible.

- Try to incorporate a wide variety of whole grains, legumes and other high-quality vegetarian sources of protein and minerals into your diet.

- Look for recreational games, sports or even workout classes that you enjoy both socially and physically. Try to fit these into your schedule a few times a week.

When we break up instinctual eating into smaller concepts, it does seem more manageable. As a busy working mom doing my best to raise three teenagers in as healthy a way as possible, I completely understand the daily challenges that can derail this type of lifestyle. On many days I do not eat a wide variety of vegetables, so I take a supplement that allows me to still get an optimal amount of these nutrients. My family does not love eating fish, so we may have this only once a week; again, I can easily supplement with a high-quality fish oil to make up for what I am missing. I am also incredibly fortunate to live in a large city that provides me and my family with additional options of healthy prepared food, including delicious vegetarian options, that are available for takeout.

These strategies all help to make instinctual eating possible, and in my personal case it is never perfect. I love many of the fast-food options that most human beings do. French fries, pizza, doughnuts and chocolate enter our home on a weekly basis. However, we do not eat this food the majority of the time; it is reserved for "special occasions" when the house is filled with other teenagers or when we are simply too exhausted to even think about preparing any type of food ourselves. I never feel bad about these types of digressions—they are simply a real part of our busy lifestyle, and all we can strive to do is take very small steps to improve, when we have the time and resolve to do it.

TRAINING TOOL: Instinctual Eating

I believe that instinctual eating leads you to a healthy relationship with your food. Part of this is about understanding and appreciating where your food comes from and who prepared it for you. Picture the difference between making soup from scratch and opening a can. To make your own, you start with bones that you boil to make a delicious broth, and then you add fresh vegetables that you sourced locally or maybe even grew in your own garden. Then you add a protein from a local butcher, or organic lentils, or possibly some leftovers from your previous night's dinner. Picture the flavours from this soup coming together on your stove as you slowly boil and mix your favourite ingredients and the delicious aroma fills your home.

Now think about a can of soup that you purchased at the store. It will usually be exceedingly high in sodium (this is where the addictive taste comes from) and extremely low in fresh, quality ingredients. It will probably also contain added sugar, to again try to trick your brain into craving it. You open the can, dump the soup in the pot and start eating within five minutes.

Now, it is important to ask yourself: Which soup will you enjoy more? Which soup do you think will provide your body with more nutrients? Which soup will you feel more satisfied with? The answers are obvious. It is equally obvious that instinctual eating is not possible without some effort and planning. I do promise, however, that if you make this effort, the results will be worth it—for both your physical and mental well-being.

RECOMMENDED READING: *Salt, Sugar, Fat: How the Food Giants Hooked Us* by Michael Moss

15

Once We Know Better... Then What?

To run with the wolf was to run in the shadows,
the dark ray of life, survival and instinct.
A fierceness that was both proud and lonely,
a tearing, a howling, a hunger and thirst . . .
A strength that would die fighting, kicking,
screaming, that wouldn't stop until the last
breath had been wrung from its body.

O.R. MELLING

I HAVE DEVOTED MOST of my life to studying and understanding human movement and how simple variations can cause improvements and challenges or sometimes pain and injury. Although I am not a neuroscientist, during university I did dissect and study the human brain. Training neuronal pathways effectively is an extremely important part of success in movement. The easiest way for me to understand brain function is to picture our brain as a series of pathways. Neurons become specialized for various patterns and they create areas of the brain designated for specific functions. I do believe that there are some differences between individuals, and certainly there are differences related to the stimulus our environment provides as we grow and develop specialized skill sets. I have transferred this understanding of neuronal pathways into my opinion that instincts are inherited neuronal patterns that our brain formed during our early development, possibly even some pathways that we were born with.

These neuronal pathways are beautifully illustrated when children are learning to crawl, grab objects, walk and eventually talk. In most cases, no one is coaching them to learn these things, or trying to explain to them to use their opposite arm and leg when crawling. Somehow that pattern is already present, and our human brain can refine this pattern or hopefully even enhance it through practice and repetition. When I was in a coffee shop having lunch, a toddler in a snowsuit wandered over and was working his way onto a couch directly across from me. I was fascinated as I observed him first tentatively feel the couch (possibly for safety), and then he pitched his head forward in an attempt to claw his way onto the couch. One of the reasons I found this movement so interesting is that toddlers' heads are by far the heaviest parts of their body, so it made perfect biomechanical sense for him to attempt his "couchsurfing" in this way. I also love the fact that no one teaches toddlers these movements, they just do them. Sometimes they have success and sometimes they fail, usually by falling over. If they are given the time and freedom to experiment, they will try again. Toddlers' movements are interesting to observe from an instinctual point of view because they probably have not yet developed the cognitive awareness of why they are doing what they are doing. They mostly explore and go with what feels right.

Although we do not have a complete understanding of the brain and all its remarkable abilities, we do learn more every day, and I believe that, as our technology in radiology allows us to observe various parts of the brain in real time, as a person is thinking about certain things or completing specific tasks, we will gain a better understanding of what drives we are born with and what instincts develop as a result of our environment.

Some days, even though health and fitness are basically my life, I feel that my efforts are inadequate in the context of the images and videos I am bombarded with daily through advertising and social media. I can rationally understand that this feeling is exactly what the advertisers are looking for. My frustration with this industry arises from the fact that I completely understand how millions of people must be feeling this same way, every single day. The invasion of social media into our daily lives only intensifies this constant feeling that we are not enough—not fit enough, not attractive enough, not popular enough, not fashionable enough. We are exposed to endless testimonials or sponsored content that tells us that if we just try this "new" workout regime, or buy the hottest piece of equipment, our life will be forever changed for the better.

The health, fitness and diet industry in North America is worth $100 billion, and when you take a step back to look at the basics, you will understand that the only way it can continue this way is if people do not get the results they are promised. I always ask this question to clients and patients: "If even one of those highly marketed diets worked in the way it promised, how big would the diet industry be?" In my mind the answer is that this "machine" of marketing, fear mongering and selling would be drastically reduced to almost zero. If there was a diet that worked, everyone would go on that diet and have wonderful results—end of story. We all know that is not the case. Diets are often plagued with temporary results; workout fads are usually the same or, worse, can lead to serious, long-lasting injuries. All of these undesirable results have another very common effect that no one ever talks about: they make people feel bad about themselves, they decrease confidence, and that feeling often leads to more spending as we try to fill the hole of inadequacy. The vicious cycle repeats itself.

I have always been fascinated by these phenomena and, to be perfectly honest, often frustrated. I am sure many of you have had the experience of your parents, out of pure enthusiasm for what you do, referring you to some crazy idea that is related to your field of study or expertise. Or a friend suggests you try a new workout regime because Gwyneth Paltrow has posted about the "magical" benefits. In the back of my mind, I think, "I have not one, not two, but *three* university degrees related to this topic, I have many years of successful experience working in this exact field, and you are suggesting I should go with the advice of a celebrity who has no actual training or education in this!" Even though I do secretly love Gwyneth, I am often amazed at how powerful the draw toward another human being can be, and how, even though you may not logically agree with what they are saying, you can easily override those thoughts with your emotions. I have realized that there must be something more to this concept

Understanding the connection between our brain, our habits, our instincts and our behaviours is essential.

_____

that I do not understand on a logical or even scientific level. This is part of the reason I became fascinated with instinct and drive theory, because I know that my parents, friends, patients and clients are very smart people. This then leads logically to the question: Why are their choices related to health, nutrition and exercise sometimes verging on ridiculous?

The other remarkable part of this behaviour is that it can repeat itself many times throughout one person's lifetime. When it comes to our health, diet and workout routines, we often do not learn from our previous mistakes. Instead, we blame the failure on our own inability to remain disciplined, or our own perceived weaknesses. I have heard many times from patients and clients that they were disappointed they did not have the willpower to stick to their diet, or that they were just not in good-enough shape to keep up with a new workout trend. Rarely is there a logical thought process that indicates to us that these new trendy routines were destined to fail.

This leads me to believe that these types of choices are not logic-driven or based on facts or science; there must be other important variables at play. However, as a health care provider and fitness expert, when I am speaking to someone about these issues or presenting a segment on television or doing a radio interview, I always quote facts and science. That is my "go-to move," that is my educational training, and it is my absolute comfort zone. The important question is, am I speaking the best language for my clients, patients or audience? The answer is, probably not.

To be ultimately successful in altering our habits or improving our lifestyle, using the same techniques we have always used may not be the road to success. Many recent studies in the health science field are supporting this same conclusion. If we want to influence our behaviour and make healthy choices, we have probably been using techniques that are not highly effective in our current lifestyle. When we look at the rising rates of obesity, cardiovascular illness and depression, the data indicates that what we have tried in the past is not working well. I believe this is because we are ignoring our basic instinctual patterns and behaviours, and in many instances we are working against these patterns instead of trying to work with them. Essentially, we are trying to alter our physical body while at the same time desperately trying to ignore our brain and those instinctual patterns we have developed over a lifetime.

Current research in an area called implementation intentions indicates that to alter health behaviours permanently, we need to focus more on psychology and behaviour and less on specific diets and exercise programs. In a meta-analysis of 26 studies related to implementation intentions, researchers found that there is enough supporting evidence to suggest that these techniques are effective enough to cause actual positive behaviour changes in health. Scientists at the Ottawa Hospital Research Institute found this research so compelling that they are now planning to implement a new technique called a "Brain Hack," directly modelled on implementation intentions. The research strategy is to improve healthy behaviours across large populations, including various groups of patients, by altering their health habits through specific Brain Hack techniques. Because the research indicates that the results are real but the changes are small in nature, the best strategy for the health of Canadians is to try to achieve small results in large populations. This is exciting, because finally someone is trying something new to solve an old and persistent problem, as opposed to developing a new drug or changing our food guide recommendations. Understanding the connection between our brain, our habits, our instincts and our behaviours is essential to nurturing our ability to make small changes that will improve our health, our performance and ultimately our happiness over a lifetime.

TRAINING TOOL: Habits

Recognizing that our behaviours and habits reflect complex neural pathways developed over a lifetime, we must also acknowledge that any type of quick fix or simple solution is not the best strategy for significantly changing the way we live our life. Small changes or Brain Hacks seem to be one promising solution. I have also found some inspiring information in a book by James Clear called *Atomic Habits*. This is one of my favourite quotes from this insightful author:

> Our genes do not eliminate the need for hard work. They clarify it. They tell us *what* to work hard on. Once we realize our strengths, we know where to spend our time and energy. We know which types of opportunities to look for and which types of challenges to avoid. The better we understand our *nature*, the better our strategy can be.

I would include our instincts in Clear's description of our "genes" and our "nature." As you will remember from the previous chapters explaining many of these direct influences on our behaviour and actions, we will find more success if we work *with* our instincts and not *against* them.

RECOMMENDED READING: *Atomic Habits: An Easy & Proven Way to Build Good Habits & Break Bad Ones* by James Clear

16

Summary of Our Human Instincts

We are conscious co-creators in the evolution of life. We have free will. And we have choices. Consequently our success is based on our choices, which are, in turn, totally dependent on our awareness.

BRUCE H. LIPTON

IF YOU BELIEVE, as I do, that we are currently living a life where we have a myriad of choices presented to us every single day, it then follows, as the chapter-opening quote explains, that "our success is based on our choices." And if that is true, then developing an enhanced awareness of why we are driven to choose the things we do should serve us well.

The author of this quote, Bruce Lipton, began his career as a cell biologist credited with many astounding scientific breakthroughs in the areas of cell membrane research. His research published in *Science* and other world-renowned journals was summarized in several best-selling books. Lipton's scientific focus shifted into an area called epigenetics, and he lives by the theory that our thoughts and intentions will have significant impacts on our health and physiology on a cellular level.

If we would like to alter the structure of our life, to enhance our instincts and ultimately be able to make better choices on a regular basis, we should also focus on the "why" and "how," as this additional information can be helpful to us in our everyday lives. How do we unlock more potential for performance, health and happiness through a better understanding of our instincts and their impact on our behaviours?

The search to "unlock" a better understanding of human consciousness is not a new pursuit; philosophers have been dedicating their lives to this quest for more than two millennia. An oft-quoted book on this subject, *The Use of Life* by John Lubbock, was first published in 1894. I reread parts of Lubbock's book as I was researching this book, and I was amazed by the similarity between some of the concepts and ideas he was talking about and the ideas and theories I was writing about over a century later, living in an environment that was completely different from his on every level. Notions like "Eat to live, but do not live to eat" have a different meaning in a culture dominated by obesity and excessive eating practices, but somehow the quote still works. Or his thoughts on the topic of rest:

> Rest is not idleness, and to lie sometimes on the grass under trees on a summer's day, listening to the murmur of the water, or watching the clouds float across the blue sky, is by no means a waste of time.

This idea still fits perfectly within the topic of rest, recovery and meditation as discussed in chapter 12. I am also inspired by Lubbock's words as he talks about "why" we should care to improve ourselves and understand more:

> Our ambition should be to rule ourselves, the true kingdom for each one of us; and true progress is to know more, and be more, and be able to do more.

As recently as the 2020 US presidential election, while Barack Obama was campaigning for the Democratic Party, he gave one of his most compelling speeches at a drive-in rally in Pennsylvania, in which he lamented the divisive politics that were dominating the election. In this speech he referred to "the better angels of our nature," a quote originally made famous by Abraham Lincoln:

We are not enemies, but friends. We must not be enemies. Though passion may have strained, it must not break our bonds of affection. The mystic chords of memory... will yet swell the chorus of the Union, when again touched, as surely they will be, by the better angels of our nature.

This is a beautiful description of an idea about our human instincts that has been discussed previously. Sometimes we listen to our "better angels" and these behaviours drive us to act in ways that benefit humanity, or even just those within our inner circle. Sometimes we make choices or behave in ways that are dictated by greed or fear. We might explain away these actions by thinking, "I had no choice" (survival instinct), or it could be a lack of experience, knowledge or often awareness. But as Barack Obama and Abraham Lincoln realized, understanding the incredible influences of "our nature" will ultimately guide us to better, kinder and less divisive choices.

It is now up to you to decide how you will use this information to improve your awareness of the choices you make, both good and bad. At various points in our life we need to take a step back and look at the overall path we have chosen, or in most cases the various paths. This sense of awareness or heightened level of consciousness seems to be unique to humans, when we compare our behaviours to those of animals. As we enter a new era that promises to be dominated by technology, along with our common "more is better" and "faster is better" attitudes, it will be more important than ever to listen to what our instincts are telling us as we decide what our new lifestyle will look like.

The well-known song "Amazing Grace" has a complicated story behind it. The original words were written in 1772 by John Newton. The story goes that after narrowly surviving a shipwreck, he felt that his life should have a "higher" purpose. So he quit his work in shipping and the slave trade and became an Anglican minister.

As we enter a new era that promises to be dominated by technology, it will be more important than ever to listen to what our instincts are telling us.

———————

Newton went on to write hundreds more hymns, sometimes translated from his weekly church sermons. Later in life he became a very vocal and influential opponent of the slave trade around the world. The hymn "Amazing Grace" is one of the most recognizable pieces of music ever written, and it has had many revivals since the original version was first put to music. It became an anthem of the American Civil War in the 1860s, and then again during the Vietnam War and the folk music movement of the 1960s. And in 2020, "Amazing Grace" became a symbol of unity and hope during the pandemic, with the legendary folksinger Judy Collins participating in the recording of a version aimed at inspiring new audiences all over the world. Although I am not a religious person, I still find that certain performances of this song bring me an overwhelming feeling of awe at our collective humanity and how far we have come.

Ultimately, in my opinion, the song is talking about choices. If we plan to live a life with amazing grace, our choices that lead to greed, hate and destruction will not get us there.

As I listened to the latest "pandemic" version of this song and read about John Newton's eventful history, the first verse took on a deep meaning:

Amazing Grace, how sweet the sound
That saved a wretch like me.
I once was lost, but now I am found.
Was blind, but now I see.

How is it possible that words written in 1772 still resonate with humankind in 2020? In the introduction of this book, there was a quote about "dust[ing] off our instincts." I relate this concept to the line in Newton's song "was blind, but now I see." We know that Newton was never literally blind, but he felt that the way he was living his life was blind to his real purpose. We might also assume that by deciding to leave the world of the slave trade and instead dedicate his life to a higher purpose, he became a happier and probably healthier person.

We have talked about instincts and their ability to enhance your health and performance, and ultimately your happiness. By developing our awareness of how our instincts work and how we can utilize this inner power to improve our life, we can hopefully make better choices for each specific area of our life. Our choices, opportunities and environments may all be unique, but our instincts have similar influences in different environments, because at one point, thousands of years ago, these patterns were developed for all human beings in a physiologically similar way.

In Part Two of this book, I am very excited to present intimate interviews with various "high-performing" individuals representing a wide spectrum of expertise and experience. I searched out actual "performers"—scientists, artists and even one of the country's top divorce lawyers—to try to better understand how these people instinctively manage in their lives and how they perceive the impact of their own instincts. I am sure you will find their answers and lessons as compelling as I did.

Below is a grouping of the instincts we looked at in the previous chapters. Obviously, there is overlap, but I hope this structure allows you to better understand the practical ways you can use your own instincts to enhance each area of your life.

INSTINCTS FOR HEALTH	INSTINCTS FOR PERFORMANCE	INSTINCTS FOR HAPPINESS
• Survival instincts (food, water, danger avoidance)	• Greed instincts	• Connection instincts
• Recovery and rest instincts	• Physical performance instincts	• Communication instincts
• Procreation instincts	• Movement instincts	• Instincts to be inspired
• Maternal and paternal instincts	• Leadership and learning instincts	• Instincts and nature
• Instinctual eating	• Communication instincts	• Attraction instincts
• Movement instincts	• Instincts for efficiency	
• Instincts and nature		

PART TWO

THE
INTERVIEWS

WHY INTERVIEWS?

WHEN I BEGAN writing this book, I gathered as much information about human instincts as I could find. Every so often, I would read something about instincts and psychology, or instincts and human movement, or even instincts in animals, and it would remind me of someone I knew or had heard of who was an expert in that particular area. I started to picture myself seeking out these experts and asking for their opinions on the interesting, exciting and sometimes even confusing ideas I was exploring. I've shortened the interviews here to focus on the book's main topics of health, happiness and performance. You can read the complete interviews at yourbetterinstincts.com.

Few things in life are more rewarding than taking an idea or concept that you are excited about and talking about it with someone you admire. That is exactly what these interviews allowed me to do. I hope you enjoy them as much as I did.

These interviews have been edited for length and clarity.

—

Stephen
Grant

Instinct is not always the best
"overall" guide to your life's conduct.
You must somehow find the
balance between thoughts and feelings.

STEPHEN GRANT

STEPHEN GRANT has been a practising lawyer for approximately 45 years, and is well known as one of Canada's top divorce lawyers. Along with his counsel practice, he acts as a mediator/arbitrator. He has received prestigious awards and medals for his extensive contributions to his profession: the Law Society Medal in 2006, the Advocates' Society Medal in 2017 and, most recently, the 2017 OBA Award for Excellence in Family Law.

Stephen is an experienced traveller and an expert on all types of art, and he has continued with a decades-long passion of trying to uncover every detail related to drinking great wines from all over the world. He has even published books and newspaper articles on these topics. I was excited to talk to Stephen about human instincts related to connection and attachment. Stephen summed it all up when he said, "Hobbies and passions can only take you so far. Human connections are critical to overall happiness."

What does the word "instinct" mean to you?

It is the same as when I am looking at my cat. He acts by instinct. He is on the table right now. Some instinct made him want to come close to me, so he jumped on the table, which he should not do, but we are not very good at making him behave! [Laughs.] He can do what he wants. In a similar way, people have an instinct to react to one another in any given situation.

Why do you think the human instinctual drive to connect with other humans can sometimes lead us down a bad path in our lives?

Because instinct is not always the best "overall" guide to your life's conduct. You must somehow find the balance between thoughts and feelings. Thoughts and feelings are not always the same things. In fact, sometimes your head and your heart do not always tell you the same thing. When that happens, it creates conflict. When you act on one as opposed to the other, you can end up in disastrous situations, and many people do.

In this book, I write about the importance of *understanding* that you have these instincts before you unthoughtfully act on them. Do you agree with that idea?

It is key! That is absolutely key. The important thing is to figure out which one, your head or your heart, is the most important. If you can mesh the two, then you can try to ensure that they are acting in concert for your best self.

In your career, I am sure you observe many relationships that have ended because of an affair, or one person cheating on another. Why do you think this happens?

I think that relationships, whether by design or inertia, do not go looking for affairs. I think affairs happen when your radar is down. If your radar is up and you are in a stable, intact relationship, people do not go looking for extramarital affairs, unless they are "players," but I am not really counting those types of people in this explanation. Affairs sometimes happen to people who are not quite looking for them, but they also do not have their radar working to prevent them.

When these things happen—a relationship breaks down or a marriage ends up in divorce—have you made any observations about what this does to a person's overall health? We can assume that a divorce is bad for someone's mental health, but have you also noticed changes in people's physical health as a result of a relationship breakdown?

Sure! If you are the person who has been cheated on, I sometimes see people practically wasting away. I see people in extreme physical distress. However, you also see people who are the perpetrators of that problem getting on with their lives in a different way.

What do you think a successful lifetime connection to a spouse or partner would look like?

I have two rules of marriage:

1 Sandy [Stephen's wife] is always right, even when she is not.
2 Whatever Sandy wants is fine with me, even when it is not!

[Sandy was also in the kitchen during our Zoom interview and she came over to say hi to me after Stephen shared this brilliant insight, and we all had a good laugh.]

Even though Sandy is here, these answers are true, and it takes a secure guy to know this. I can tell you this, though: affairs are not always the particular causes of marriage breakdowns. They are the symptoms of a bigger problem, such as growing apart, unhappiness or personal sadness, or when someone is unhappy with themselves. These situations can happen to both women and men. The other thing that has happened or that I have noticed over my 45 years of doing this is that women are much more inclined to have affairs than they used to be. It used to be mostly men, but now there are way more women that come into my practice that have had affairs.

You have also been able to explore art, poetry, travel, food and wine. You have even written books on some of these things. How important are these passions to your overall happiness?

They are critical. They are essential. It is part of the spiritual mélange right now. Not everyone has a particular passion. I have friends who joke with me about my varied interests, but it is really a life force and life-affirming for me. If I did not have that, I might be lying in bed all day, feeling dreadfully sorry for myself. The point is that hobbies and passions can only take you so far. Human connections are critical to overall happiness.

Chris Hadfield

You do not have time to change your unthinking reaction, which is basically your instinct. It is the same when playing guitar.

CHRIS HADFIELD

COLONEL CHRIS HADFIELD was the first Canadian commander of the International Space Station. Commander Hadfield's ability to inspire and educate so many of us about space, science and even music is what makes him such a unique and iconic person. He has co-created and hosted several television shows, is the author of three internationally bestselling books, and has even recorded an album, *Space Sessions: Songs from a Tin Can*.

Today, Chris spends time as an adjunct professor at the University of Waterloo and leads the space stream at the Creative Destruction Lab. As a highly sought-after public speaker and energetic educator, he was generous enough with his time to chat with me about human instincts, and when training takes over.

Can you recall a time in your life when you were being led by facts, or people, or circumstances in one direction but your instincts were telling you to take another direction? How did this turn out for you?

The job of a test pilot and astronaut relies little on instinct. There is not an instinctive reliance in a spaceship or during a spacewalk because you are working with really complex technical things. We all instinctively count on gravity and we expect gravity to do all kinds of things. As soon as you rely on your instincts to do what gravity always does, and you find yourself in a weightless environment, you are in big trouble. We have been fooled several times because of that. Here is a specific example.

I was building the Canadian Robot Arm, which we called Canadarm2. It was launched to the International Space Station during my second space flight, back in 2001, and it was my first spacewalk. It was also Canada's first spacewalk, and one of the things we had to do was unfold and bolt Canadarm2 together, and then raise it manually up out of the cradle. This is sort of like lifting the end of a telephone pole, if you can imagine, but where the telephone pole is attached to a big hinge at the bottom. We had thought about it, we talked about it, we sort of understood what we were doing.

But one day we were in the huge underwater swimming pool where we practise our spacewalking procedures, called the Neutral Buoyancy Laboratory. I was watching Scott Parazynski work on this, and as I was watching, something started tickling at the back of my thoughts. There is no gravity in the lab, but I realized he was back-driving a lot of gear mechanism. The arm is not just a hinge, but it also includes the gears that drive it. The thought popped into my head, "How much force is he working against there?" I asked our best technicians that day, "So how hard is that lift going to be?" They said it will be negligible, and I said, "Okay, good. How negligible?" Then they finally said, "Well, we don't really know."

One of the facts we did know was that he would be wearing a spacesuit, and that means that part of the lift is increased by the structure of your suit. If it turns out to be an exceptionally heavy lift, he runs a definite risk of popping a shoulder joint out of his suit.

It turned out that this was not a trivial question and we decided that we needed to know the answer. This is where my instinct and intuition had alerted me to the fact that maybe our logic might not be right. We eventually went down to Florida, to where the actual arm was, and bought a fish scale. We took that fish scale out to the end of the arm and we pulled to see what the actual weight would be. It turned out to be right at the absolute limit of Scott's lifting ability. The way that we had planned to do it would not work! The structure would not have been strong enough to be able to take the load. It would have blown our spacewalk. If we had not combined our instincts with our knowledge, we would have never got to the right answer.

You seem to be a data-driven, "practice makes perfect" type of person. I have listened to your TED Talks about being in space and your explanations of how you go through the procedures repeatedly. Do you find, after all your practice, that some of your movements in space would become subconscious or automatic?

Oh, absolutely! Yeah, and you need it. You do not have time to change your unthinking reaction, which is basically your instinct. It is the same when playing guitar. I know what chord is coming next, I can just feel it. Once you have made 100,000 chord changes, you then can play along with a song even if you have never heard the song before. When I was learning to fly airplanes as a young pilot, I would go and get into the airplane at night in the hangar and run through all the emergency procedures over and over again. If there's a fire and if the cockpit is filled with smoke, you must know what to reach for and instinctively what you're supposed to do next.

The term that we often use is "Bold Face," and in an aircraft operating manual there is an entire chapter on Bold Face. These are emergency procedures you must memorize because, when it happens, there isn't going to be time to look anything up. We used to say that all Bold Face is written in blood because that is the reason it got there; someone got it wrong and they died. The Bold Face represents something the crew needs to know, and they need to know it cold. Basically, you change your instinctive abilities. You have to turn your cognitive thinking into instinctive reactions.

Charles Darwin taught us that the most adaptable of the species are the most likely to survive. Throughout your life, you seem to have excelled at adapting, sometimes to very extreme environments. What do you think makes you exceptional at adapting to a particular environment?

I am purposeful. I am normally doing things for a reason; I am not just driven by pattern. Let's say you're trying to climb Mount Everest and you know that for 14 days before you go, you're staying in a crappy little hotel in Kathmandu, but hey, you're climbing Everest, so you don't really care. Or maybe I am at Everest base camp and it is cold, but if you are doing things with purpose, then the transient problems of where you happen to be right now are not nearly as important, and I think that makes you more adaptable.

I also grew up on a farm. I did not grow up in luxurious circumstances. I grew up in a kind of a rough-and-tumble, work-related, multi-kid environment and so it just was not all that important that everything had to be just so. My wife and I have been together since high school, but I was in the military and we moved about 25 times. The "place" is just where you are right now, and you should not get too worried about it.

I am also much more interested in the future than I am in the past. What really matters is what are we going to do next, and we have got some serious problems to solve. The real fascination is in learning and changing who you are to be able to do things that you have never done before. To me, that decreases the importance of stasis. I am much more interested in becoming more capable and understanding things better in the future.

I love your optimism. It seems that you go into a challenging situation with a purpose but also with some optimism that everything will work out well.

If you put me in any airplane in the world, blindfolded me and put it into an inverted spin with one engine failed, and then handed it to me—that is a solvable problem. But boy, when I was 14, if you had done that to me, I would have died. So, it's not really optimism, it's more pragmatism based on proven ability.

I am not falsely optimistic. For example, I play music a lot and if I am going to be playing with a symphony, that is a big deal! There are all those people and there is no way to go back. You must get your cue and you must get the chords right and all the rest of it. I practise, and I visualize, and I anticipate, and I try and change who I am so that in the moment I can give the impression of being optimistic. I am ready, and it is way easier to be optimistic if you are prepared and if you have a plan.

Where do you find the inspiration to develop your skills and talents to such a high level in so many vastly different areas? For example, you are an expert in science, math, space travel, music and even photography.

I think everybody should be perpetually dissatisfied with their skill sets. If you say to yourself, "I don't need to get any better at that," well then, you never will. In fact, you are probably going to get worse at it, because you're going to get rusty. Look at any hockey player after a two-month layoff. If you are not trying to improve who you are, then you're going to get worse. You are going to decay, you are going to become a rusted piece of metal. You get one real go-around, and we are limited by the time of our lifespan.

My wife is completing her fourth university degree right now. She has been a computer programmer and systems analyst. Then she was a professional chef, and she ran a roofing company. Now she runs our company, and she is also back at university studying fine arts, design and ceramics—and why wouldn't you? What else are you going to do—watch cat videos?

Let's say you play guitar so well that you are the best guitar player in the world. Well, in a week you might not be, someone else could come along. Gretzky is no longer the greatest hockey player in the world. We should recognize that greatness is transient, and even if you are called the greatest, well, it is going to pass soon and then you'll just be one of the hockey players.

Like everything else, you should be working on getting a little better at anything that is important to you. There is so much joy to be found in creation and creativity, in finding a way to do something better than you have ever done it before, in seeing something in a way that is different from how you have seen it before. If you go to Moscow for the first time, it is easy to feel overwhelmed because it can seem quite unfriendly, especially if you are unable to speak the language. However, if you learn to speak Russian, Moscow reveals itself to you in a completely different way, as a magnificent, interesting, thousand-year-old city full of stories, intrigue and coolness. But unless you change or adapt who you are, you will miss all of that; you are not going to get it. That is true for everything.

Try to always be questioning: "What did I accomplish at the end of the day?" Or asking yourself, "What did I learn today?" Or "My wife said something really smart today and I have got to try to remember it or internalize that." Or "I saw something that was so beautiful, like the sunrise this morning, when the sun was still below but I looked up and Mars was just above the horizon and I could see Jupiter and Saturn over to the right as the blue of the sky was starting to appear." It is just the realization of what those important moments are, what they mean and what else we will eventually discover about them.

—

Geddy
Lee

To develop a musical instinct means that you must have enough experience at failure to recognize when you have an opportunity to succeed.

GEDDY LEE

EDDY LEE is best known as the lead vocalist and bassist of the band Rush. It is not easy to capture Geddy in a simple bio, but I love what is written on the Rush website: "Musician. Chronic Collector. Baseball Geek. Fermented Grape Enthusiast."

Having had the privilege of hanging out with Geddy over many years, I would also add "Rock Star" in every sense of the word, along with fun, kind person and bestselling author. As you will read in this interview, he is so much more than the music. But let's face it, the music is pretty amazing too! This interview emphasizes that if we focus our energy on listening to our instincts for curiosity and learning, we will ultimately find true joy in that journey.

Do you think your instincts have influenced your writing and performing throughout your music career?

I think you do develop musical instinct. Again, it is a process. I do not think you are born with musical instinct; I think you are born with talent. Every person has a different capability that they are born with. For some people it is sports; some people are born with a body that gives you the possibility of succeeding and the capability of being an athlete. I think that musicians are born with a capability but then they decide whether to develop it or not. That is a whole other thing, and that is subject to conditions. Conditions are what your home life represents. It is what your educational life represents. Your cultural or social advantages or disadvantages. All those things play into your ability to develop that musical capability.

Once you understand you have that capability, you can then start to exercise that. That means you start making music. My good friend Mendelson Joe has this expression: "Make new mistakes." I think that step one in developing your musical instinct is to make those mistakes. So, you write your first song, and it is shitty. You start with that shitty song. Then the next time you write a song, you try to make it less shitty, until all the shitty things start to subside and the better parts of your talents start to show through. I think that takes years. To develop a musical instinct means that you must have enough experience at failure to recognize when you have an opportunity to succeed. That is the circumstance that goes into making your good instincts for music.

We all have an instinct for curiosity and learning, along with an instinct to be inspired. It seems that you were able to discover and understand this better than most people at an incredibly young age. You have managed to run with it, and that is inspiring.

I think there are two different issues here. On the one hand, you have an instinct, and on the other hand, you have what I would call an intuition. To me, intuition is more of an educated and cultured version of the same thing. I really see instinct as primal. When you use the term "instinct" in certain circumstances, it feels like the word should be "intuition," because you are using a database in your system that you have cultivated. When the right thing comes along, you have the idea through your education that this is the thing for you. I think there is a subtle difference between the two terms. It can be argued that an instinct is not controllable but instead it is implanted. The definition of the word is "something that you do without thinking."

You have dedicated a significant amount of your time to hiking and spending time doing activities that are connected to nature. Would you agree that your time spent in nature is good for you from a physiological standpoint?

Absolutely! I believe that is true, from a spiritual perspective. I am not a religious person. I do not believe in God, but in my own way I am a spiritual person in that I believe in nature. I believe that standing in a forest by yourself and listening to the sounds around you and smelling the ground and the blossoming trees, hearing the birds—all that connects you to Mother Nature, and that is my God. That is where I go to replenish my spirit and to lose all the grime of urban life. I do not mean just physical grime; it is the psychological grime of urban life. It starts to jam up your works. I think the best way to refresh is to be as alone as you can in nature. I am lucky that I have a partner who I adore, and who I think likes me too—and we both like the same stuff. We both like to spend our time in nature when we are not hopping around the world on airplanes. I find it very soulful and very replenishing. I think that has an impact on my body. I feel stronger, healthier, and I tend to do more exercise because I am out in a wild environment and I want to walk through it.

One of the other things I admire about you is that you seem to have a great appreciation for food and where it comes from. You also tend to prioritize the importance of connecting with your friends through food. How do food and these connections through food affect your life?

It is a particularly important aspect of my life because my social life, to a large degree, is built around the sharing of food and wine. I grew up in a household that was a survivor household. My parents were survivors from World War II. They had come over here after the war and they had old Eastern European food traditions, meaning a lot of overcooked foods, not much that was fresh. Many foods came out of a can, and my mother and father both worked, so it was not what I would call the most elevated cuisine. What I learned about food, I had to learn out and about.

As a teenager, of course, your social life revolves around your friends, usually drinking beer and passing a joint. As you get older, those things become a bit tiresome, so your social life evolves to something slightly more sophisticated, where you might meet your friends at a good restaurant. You talk about the food and you share the wine. I stopped smoking pot when I was in my late 20s, and I replaced it with sharing wine. [Laughs.] It is just a different kind of joint—we pass the bottle instead. I think that stayed with me.

—

Alex
Lifeson

*I was always the instinctive writer.
I excelled more in the spontaneous
"in the moment" ideas.
That was always my strength.*

ALEX LIFESON

ALEX LIFESON has spent a big part of his life as the lead guitarist for the band Rush, but he is so much more than a Hall of Fame musician. From the Rush website we learn he is also a "Pilot. Painter. Golfer." Alex and I have been friends for several years; still, prior to this interview, I did not know that he was driven by a creative and artistic instinct in such a spontaneous and confident way. I loved how he explained that he honours his creativity by "get[ting] out of the way of it," while at the same time he is aware that his maturity and hard-earned life experience has allowed him to use this instinct in a better way.

What does the word "instinct" mean to you?

For me, the word "instinct" describes how I have operated throughout my career as a musician. As a writing team, particularly between Geddy and me, because we started working together at such a young age [15 years old], we have gone through many different levels in our relationship. When you get a bunch of creative people together, often everyone's idea is the best. That is something, I think, you get over with maturity. Once you can establish what the actual strengths are in the team, it makes all of that much easier.

With Rush, Geddy was always much more methodical. He would want to go through all the "wrong" ideas before he would feel comfortable and confident that we had found the right idea. That was great, because that process got us to try a ton of different things and ultimately got us to the best outcome. For me, I was the opposite. I was always the instinctive writer. I excelled more in the spontaneous "in the moment" ideas. That was always my strength. When we are doing guitar solos in the studio, for example, it is typical to do multiple takes. My first few takes were always the best. Number six, seven and eight were just kind of repeats. I always had that ability.

It works the same way for me now when I am painting. [Alex paints regularly for the Kidney Foundation of Canada for their "Brush of Hope" program. The paintings are done by various artists and celebrities to be auctioned off to raise funds for the charity.] I usually just stare at the canvas for a while and then I think about what paint technique I want to use, and I start. I spent two to three weeks working on my last painting and then I decided to redo the whole painting with a fork and got rid of my brushes. After a while, I thought, "This is awful! This is the worst thing ever!" I started then adding more paint to it and then that gave me another idea and then instinctively I began building up on this other idea. In fact, there is now another painting beneath the finished painting! That would probably not happen for me if I were not that sort of person—if I was not a spontaneous, instinctive person. Sometimes I am a little too instinctive and I become a bit emotional too quickly. Over the years, I have learned to understand those feelings a bit better, and that helps the whole process.

When you were performing with Rush, before you were world-famous rock stars, did you ever go into a gig and have an instinctual feeling that things might not go as well as you were hoping for? Or that you were going to have to work especially hard to win over a new crowd of fans?

Sure! Many, many, many times. We always had a confidence in what we were doing and a kind of "take it or leave it" approach. We knew that we were going to do the best that we possibly can and that is all that we are able to do. If you hate us after all that, then you hate us. That is fine. I think that is the type of attitude you need to have, but that also comes with confidence—knowing that what you are doing is honest and true to yourself. It was never really a matter of trying to please someone else. We were also fortunate to have a large fan base that respected that in us. We always stayed true to what we were doing.

When I look at all the work you have done over the years, Alex, I believe that the instinct to connect with people is extraordinarily strong within you. You are great in interviews. You have an amazing sense of humour. Where do you feel that connection instinct comes from in your life?

Everybody has a need to connect. Being a musician and having a career as a musician from my youth right through to my old age provided that kind of an arena for me. That is exactly what we would do on a nightly basis. We connect with thousands of people through music. Then there are other things such as my art, or doing an interview, whatever it might be—it becomes a normal part of your being. You do not really think about it, you just act upon it. Being creative is the same way; you don't spend time trying to figure out "Where is this coming from?" or "What is the source of my creativity?" You get out of the way of it. That has always been the most important thing, to just let it naturally happen. Be aware of it, but be almost an observer while it is happening.

This is exactly what I believe understanding your instincts allows you to do and why I think this knowledge is so important. It is like us coaching an elite athlete. During a competition or performance, you do not want to be overthinking and analyzing a bunch of things, but as you said, "get out of the way" and let your instincts take over but at the same time "be an observer," so you are aware

of what is happening. Do you think you are able to do this because of how many hours you spend practising as a musician?

Definitely! Those 10,000 hours that everyone talks about, or in our case 40,000 to 50,000 hours, are an important part of your development and your confidence and your abilities. I play much better now after not playing for a long time than I did when I was playing *all* the time and would take a short break. I was always a bit rustier and less confident after a short break on the road in the early days, even though we were playing every single night. Later on in my career, I could take a month off, pick up my guitar, and things would feel easier and I could find a better flow.

Was there a moment where your instincts caused you to take a different path and it turned out better for you and the band?

Our most pivotal moment, and this has to do with the whole band, was after we released our third record. There was a lot of concern from the record company because, although the record was important to us creatively, we were wanting to experiment with it, try out some new ideas and develop our confidence in what exactly we were trying to do, but it was not a big seller. Without that commercial success, the record company started to get worried about their investment in the band. There was a lot of pressure for us to consider remaking the first record or try to do something that would be more commercially accessible. I remember sitting in dressing rooms and in the back of the car driving around North America, talking about what we should do for the next record, and I can still feel the pressure that we were under. We ended up writing *2112*, and that became our most pivotal record. Not our biggest-selling record, but probably our most important record. We gave in to the idea that we were doing the right thing by following our creative feelings when writing the record and we would continue to do that. If it did not work out, we would just go back to whatever jobs we could find. Seriously! I was talking to my father about coming back and working in his plumbing company.

We stuck to our idea, and our instincts told us that we were doing the right thing. Sure enough, although it was not an overnight success, it took a year for that record to really make an imprint, but after that our record company trusted us. Our decision bought us our freedom and independence as musicians. It allowed us to go with our own ideas. It was a good feeling, and it started with that "gut" feeling that writing a record for commercial success was wrong. We needed to go out and make the record we believed in.

———

Dr. Deborah MacNamara

The attachment instinct is the instinct that governs human behaviour most of all.

DR. DEBORAH MACNAMARA

DR. DEBORAH MACNAMARA is a counsellor and educator for both parents and professionals. She is guided by the relational-developmental approach of Dr. Gordon Neufeld. She is also on the faculty of the Neufeld Institute.

Deborah is the author of the bestselling book *Rest, Play, Grow: Making Sense of Preschoolers (Or Anyone Who Acts Like One)* and a children's picture book, *The Sorry Plane*. She is a dynamic teacher and experienced counsellor with over 20 years' experience in educational and mental health settings. Deborah is passionate in taking developmental science and making it applicable to everyday life in the home and classroom. The underlying purpose of all her services is to *put adults in the driver's seat* by making sense of kids from the inside out. She is able to explain everyday questions, complex problems and strategies for making headway with a child or teen in terms that regular humans (without psychology Ph.D.s) understand!

I was excited to speak to Deborah about maternal and paternal instincts, but as you will read, there was so much more to be learned about so many things, from her vast experience and understanding of human behaviour to her expertise in child development. I also appreciated the sentiment that to encourage humans as a species to develop and mature both emotionally and physically, we must find our important rituals and routines that will give us space and ultimately help us find more joy in our relationships.

What do you think are the most important things for us as humans to understand about our instincts?

The instinct that drives human beings the most is the instinct for attachment—an instinct for togetherness, for connection and for deep relationships. The reason why this instinct is there in human beings, and in all mammal species, is that it aids survival by having us want to be together. It is not just about food for human beings, it is much deeper. It is about an invitation to share your feelings, an invitation to express yourself, a place of home. It should be a deep place of rest. The attachment instinct is all about survival, but not just on a physiological level. It is a part of everything for human beings, from our emotions, to how we cognitively develop, to our spirituality. It is the foundation from which all growth emanates. It is an instinct that pushes us together, and for our children what that means is that it helps them and secures the relationship so that they depend on us for the purpose of caretaking. If they are not glued to us, then it makes it exceedingly difficult to take care of a young child. I would say that the attachment instinct is *the* instinct that governs human behaviour most of all.

Do you think our current way of living, specifically in an urban "high-tech" environment, allows us to develop our instincts to their highest potential?

The way I would view that question is as follows: Does technology get in the way of our relationships and interfere with human attachment? I would say, not necessarily. It depends on how we use and govern our tools and our technology. They are more of a "quick fix" toward attachment. It is easy to go to your phone or computer for a quick depersonalized fix. I do not think technology necessarily *has* to be an issue in this way. It is a temptation, but if we develop our children's full potential for relationships—and really, that is the goal of caretaking or parenting—if we develop a sense of self, belonging, sharing and intimacy within our children, then they are less likely to be hungry for substitutes that do not really fill that need. We are often attracted and attached to other humans who have a similar level of attachment as we have.

The hungrier you are for attachment, the more likely you might be to turn to social media to fill the voids in your life. The only problem that I can see with technology is that it is a temptation, but we are exposed to all kinds of temptations. When we are feeling sad or unsupported, there are many things humans turn to in an attempt to fill those voids. Technology has just become one of the latest. The good thing about technology is that it does provide some visual contact, and it provides some auditory contact, and I think that you can get a sense of being connected.

What I look at is not the technology itself; I look at what is driving the use. If you are using it to deal with a lack and a loss in your life, then you should address that. If you are using it for a bit of entertainment and you are aware that is the case—for example, my work is done and I am going to take a break, or I just want to tune out for a bit—then you should just tune out and enjoy it. Put it in its ritual and use it properly. We should not always just blame technology for our problems.

We need to figure out how these tools fit in as a part of the ongoing industrial revolution. How do we fit them into the context of our lives, and how do we keep what is sacred, things like human attachment and the instinct to be together, preserved and protected? How do we keep those essential attachments with our children and not let our relationships get hijacked by technology used as a substitute? How do we protect the concept of "play" and ensure our children are spending time with this essential part of human development? I do not think we should demonize technology, but as a developmentalist I am more interested in what is driving the use. Does it enhance our development or is it a detour?

Can you explain how our instincts change over our lifetime? For example, it is often believed that teenaged boys can sometimes ignore their instincts for survival and are drawn to participating in riskier behaviours. How do you think our instincts and behaviours evolve as we age?

I do not think our instincts change, but I think the expression of them changes. For example, how you attach as a grandparent is different than how you attach as a parent. Instincts to attach, for survival, are essential; that never leaves us. We do become better able to function independently. Our hunger for relationship will slightly decrease as we become better able to function on our own as young adults. What I see is that the expression of the instinct changes, but it is dependent on "healthy" development. You reach a point where you can function well as a separate social person.

When we look at the end of someone's life, we observe a beautiful circle, because the expression for attachment does change. Our focus shifts to concepts of "What do I want to leave behind?" "What do I need to finish up?" Grandparents are assumed to be able to transfer into this position of elder, and when it is done in a healthy way, they can become incredible agents of healthy development for the generations to come. I believe the instinct for attachment is forever and it drives your behaviour throughout your life. What changes is how you express this instinct. A child, a parent and a grandparent will all have unique expressions of this instinct, and they will all usually have a different focus within this instinct.

The question about adolescence is interesting. What you are describing to me in this question could be a lack of an "alarm" mechanism, and I think that is driven more by our emotions. We know that our emotions are attached to our instincts, and that many times our expressions of emotions are related to our instincts. Not all teenagers are reckless and without alarm mechanisms to help them be safe and want to preserve themselves. Then we must make sense of the ones that *are* reckless. I do not think this is a "normal" behaviour. I think that sometimes society sees it as normal, but it is not natural for our feelings of alarm to leave us. That usually means that something has been muted, tuned out or inhibited. In neuroscience we know that emotional inhibition is possible, and that it is often driven by our instinct for attachment. For example, if we looked at a group of teenagers about to embark on a risky activity, and if you felt that if you did *not* participate in this activity, it would cost you your relationship or your "attachment" to this group, your brain may inhibit your alarm to preserve the connection. But if you are with a peer group that celebrates differences, and that wants everyone to be their "own" person, then you would probably feel safer to step away from the group and say, "I am not doing what the rest of you are doing; I do not feel comfortable."

When we talk about risky behaviour in teens, or anybody, my first questions would be, "Where have their tears gone?" or "Where has their caring gone? Why is their alarm so muted?" We do know that teens go through a period of idealism that prepares the path for them to become a separate human being, but they do still need guardrails on to help. Instincts and emotions mostly operate at the level of unconscious, and to be able to use them we need to bring them into consciousness, but this won't be possible if emotional defences are in operation. The interesting thing about adolescents is that because their brains are under so much strain from the large amounts of changes going on, there are studies that show, if you bring a bunch of them together, they sometimes have so much going on that they can become overwhelmed emotionally, so that they are operating at the level of a preschooler. This is when we often see them make errors in judgment. This could be a temporary thing, because they happen to be emotionally overwhelmed in the moment, or it can be part of a bigger problem, where they are muted emotionally. These issues may also not be permanent, but simply because of too much going on for them to process.

Do you think there is a similar response with addiction, where the drugs or the chemicals cause a muted emotional response to various dangers in life?

Yes, I agree with that. If we look at addiction, we should always be asking, "What is the void that cannot be tolerated that is underneath the addiction?" I would come from the place that there has been a loss, or a lack, or a significant void, that for whatever reason could not be grieved, held on to, could not be put into words, that we could not find our tears about, and then "things" are used to fill that void. That can be said for any addiction, it does not have to be a substance; it could be television, technology or even food. We use all sorts of things to fill this "lack."

When we are not released from our attachment hunger, we sit in a void. The question then becomes: "When the void opens up, what goes in it? Can we put words in it? Does our play carry us through it? Can we seek expression? Can we find our tears? Is there a recognized vulnerability there? Is there support from another person?" So many people lose their tears because as children we find no one there to support them. It was not safe to have tears. How could you find your tears when you got in trouble for them, or if you were not allowed to feel frustrated? It was all about survival. When your very baseline survival is in question, your emotions, expressions and awareness of them become a complete luxury. There is no processing trauma in these types of situations. Gordon Neufeld put this really well when he said, "There is nothing more addictive than something that almost works." That is what keeps you on the hook! You get a fix. You find temporary relief from the pain, and the anguish, and where the emotions from the lacks and the losses sit, and then you hang on to that substitute because it provides temporary relief. That feeling then has the ability to take you out of the orbit of the things that you actually need to survive or the things that really fulfill you.

The more you work for love, the less you can rest in it. That is my feeling on addiction. When we give people the place and community to feel supported, and they feel the space to be themselves and they feel held on to as they are, there is a generous invitation. They are transformed. They become different people, and that is the path to recovery. With addiction there are many soothing substitutes, but they do not satiate you.

Tracy
Moore

Instinct is about acting based on your gut—using that thing that is inside all of us, but really *listening to it.*

TRACY MOORE

TRACY MOORE is the host of Canada's longest-running life-style show, *Cityline*. She has been on *Hello!* magazine's "Most Beautiful" list, carried the torch for the Pan Am Games, threw the first pitch at a Toronto Blue Jays game, hosted Citytv's Grammys red carpet show, and twice a year designs her own fashion line, Tracy Moore by Freda's. After the show, Tracy can be found on her living room rug in a heated game of Uno with her husband, Lio; her kids, Sidney and Eva; and her fur baby, Ozzie. Tracy says being a mother is hands down her biggest accomplishment to date.

I have had the pleasure of working with Tracy as an expert on her show, and I am always in awe of her intelligence, passion and curiosity and how she is able to wrap all those qualities together while at the same time understanding that laughter is the best connector. There is never a time that I am with Tracy when I am not laughing about something, but also feeling her kindness through it all. We laughed a lot during this interview.

What does the word "instinct" mean to you?

Instinct is about acting based on your gut—using that thing that is inside all of us, but *really* listening to it. I think that is the gap that a lot of us fall into sometimes. We all have it, we all feel instinct, we just do not always listen to it.

Let's go back a decade or so to when you were a news reporter. What skills or attributes do you think helped you shift your career so successfully and move it into a major positive trajectory?

It was not an easy transition, going from news, where you were supposed to try to be as objective and fact-based as possible. Then, moving into the lifestyle space, everybody wanted to know what I fed my baby for breakfast, what my husband did for a living, where did I buy my blouse. Immediately, I became the story. I then had to figure out, how do I still be "me" but on television? It took a while to get that.

Not only was I learning the format of lifestyle television, but I was also not a lifestyle television watcher. This was not where I had planned my life to be going—I wanted to be Diane Sawyer. If not that, I was going to be a foreign news correspondent. First I had to learn what the format was, and then I had to go out there every single day with people who vocalized that they did not want to see me and kept asking, "When is the previous host coming back?" It really was a lot of humility. I was so excited to have the opportunity. I decided to not focus on the negative emails or the critiques. I knew I just needed some time. I really hoped that Canada and my bosses would just give me the time.

I am a fast learner. I had to put my ego aside and ask for help and look for information and lean on people who were smarter than me, then build my comfort and confidence. The only way you build confidence is by doing the same thing over and over and over again. Thank goodness I was able to have some time to ease into the role. It probably took me a good 18 months to feel comfortable with the format. Then it was a matter of, how do I fit who I am into what the show is? That took *many* more years.

Was there a time in your life when facts or people were telling you to do something a certain way, or go in a certain direction in your life, but your instincts were telling you the opposite? What did you do, and how did things turn out?

When I first took over *Cityline*, everyone told me I was "too nice," saying things like, "You are being bossed around, we need you to find your bitch pants," "You need to take charge," "Start coming in two guns a-blazing." I had so much unsolicited advice from all sorts of people basically from everywhere. I thought to myself, "This is so not who I am!" I would come home to my husband and ask him, "Do you think I need to be more forceful?" He would say, "No, you are learning. You need to learn how to do this thing before you start bossing people around!" I would even get it from my bosses in meetings, when I would agree with them. They would then say, "You are too nice."

It was a very stressful situation, but I felt very secure in the idea that I know who I am and I do not need to walk into a room and bang my fists on a table to get decisions to be made. I would rather collaborate. I would like to hear what everyone has to say. I like to be fair about things. Leaders can lead with soft skills, and I would say that I stuck with what felt right to me instinctually, and I feel like I am reaping the benefits of that now, because I have always stayed true to who I am. I have even had a lot of people try to tell the world who I am when it is not true, and anyone who knows me knows that. It comes from always being true to who I am, and I am very happy that I never tried to become something else.

You are an expert connector. What do you think allows you to form genuine and real connections with people, sometimes very quickly?

I do not love small talk. One of the great things I have found from working on television is that when I bump into people, there is immediate familiarity. I might be at a grocery store and someone will come right up to me and start talking to me as if we know each other. I kind of like that, because what happens is, when we start talking, we quickly go from "I didn't know you shopped here!" to "My husband is unemployed" or "I have just had a miscarriage and you had a segment on the show about this." I love when interactions are intimate like that. We can be talking about sex, menopause, our hairy legs and armpits—all of that stuff can happen backstage within two minutes of seeing each other. I love that we can get to the essence of things quickly.

For me, it is about "I see Stacy and you are not just the chiropractor/fitness expert, you are a person!" Then I want to connect on a human level about whatever is happening in your life and whatever is happening in your world. It does not always work that way. When I spoke with Victoria Beckham, there were too many walls up, too many people involved, so much security—so much of that stuff that interferes with a genuine connection. But for most celebrities, even someone like Matthew McConaughey—I just interviewed him about his new book—I saw him trying to connect to the Zoom and he was squinting and I looked at him and said, "Your eyes are taking a hit from COVID, aren't they?" and he basically yelled, "Yessss! I am on these screens all frigging day!" At that moment, it does not matter that he is a star, what matters is that he is a human, and we are all going through this experience together of trying to survive all the screen time and trying to keep our mental health together! I feel that we should all be having fun here, and if we can have a real connection, everyone at home will feel and see a real connection too!

Our instincts to survive are some of the most powerful drivers of human behaviour, and as I have followed your amazing work through the Black Lives Matter movement, I sometimes would see ridiculous comments written to you as a response to your efforts. I worry that some days the stress from this would be overwhelming and you would need to draw upon your survival instincts just to get up the next day and work some more. What do you think allowed you to keep going, or gave you the energy and resolve?

I felt a couple of things. I did feel a sense of urgency, and I do not know if that was real or imagined. I had spent a lifetime not being able to have these difficult conversations outside of my community. Any time I would dip my toe into something race related, I would be afraid of getting an answer that was going to be ignorant and then I might have to re-evaluate my relationship with that person. I could also be in a situation where folks would be overly sensitive, and I would have to spend the rest of the conversation placating them or trying to make them feel better. Basically, I had just stopped talking about it, outside of the black community. Suddenly, people were asking me to talk about it, so I really felt there was a timer on, and then there was going to be a "Time's up!" I wanted to try my best to get some substantive change happening.

It is great to see "Black Lives Matter" spray-painted on the street, but I really wanted to see actual changes. For example, is Rogers Media going to change their hiring processes? I was thinking, "What can *Cityline* do for this? Can we make some decisions right now that are going to last beyond people's appetite for talking about this thing?" I felt pressure, and that was part of the reason I kept going.

The second part of this answer is that I had to rest. I had to take breaks. I felt that I was being beaten down in a way that I had not really been a part of before. I had never had so many people understand these absolute truths about me, and I felt that some people were upset about these truths. It was like they were opening their eyes and saying, "Well, she is not just nice, she is saying that racism exists—and that hurts me." When I saw these comments, some from intelligent people, some from people who just do not know, I would be lying if I said that they did not hurt. I felt that I was not saying anything against anyone. I was truthfully speaking about experience and trying to use this moment to educate. It really did bother me that even by opening my mouth, some people felt threatened enough to tell me to "just shut up."

What I then found was that there were many people who were sending me messages and saying, "I do not feel that you are okay right now." They would suggest that maybe things were getting to be a bit too much. They *saw* it! These people could still see that I was getting beaten down. The beautiful part of the story is that I had so many people reach out. They sent me gifts, they sent me helpful advice, they even encouraged me to take a break.

As parents, we have developed extraordinarily strong maternal instincts to protect our children and help them grow in every way in a healthy, safe environment. What do you hope for when you work toward the future for your family and for Sidney and Eva?

There is such a wide variety these days with how people are structuring the lives of their children and managing expectations—or not. There is the group that sets very high expectations, where a B average is unacceptable, and the kids are expected to, at the very least, complete a university undergraduate degree. I get that. My kids have so many resources that they can tap into. They have two parents with master's degrees. You and your husband are in a similar situation. We look at our kids and we think, "We give you *everything*! You should be able to perform."

Honestly, I think this pandemic has changed so much about how I am seeing success. Of course, there is a part of me that wants my children to be successful. I would love for them to find something that they are passionate about and be able to turn that into something. But at the end of the day, I really need them to be happy. The focus that I have right now on my mental health, I am passing that on to my kids! I need to know that Eva is not driving herself crazy because she was late getting into her Google Classroom. I worry that she puts too much pressure on herself, and I heard her crying this morning because everyone was on their final copy of something and she was still on her second rough draft. These things cannot be the things that take you out. I want them to learn what their tools will be in their tool box to keep themselves happy. If that is two dog walks a day, arranging to see their friends at the park, whatever it is, I want them to have access to those tools. I mostly need them to be happy. I want them to learn how to tweak their brain and their body so that they feel good about life. That is it!

—

Matt
Nichol

That feeling of competition and wanting to win is part of our instinctual drive . . . It is always there.

MATT NICHOL

MATT NICHOL is a veteran strength and conditioning coach who has trained professional and elite amateur athletes since the late 1990s, working with numerous individuals and teams. Matt is an industry leader who hosts Canada's premier summer off-season hockey camp for top NHL players. Every year, 25 NHL players and 25 of the best amateur players get accepted into the program. Using the latest technology, equipment and scientific research, Matt tailors training and nutritional plans to maximize his athletes' performance.

Outside of his work with professional athletes and Olympians, sports teams and athletic associations, Matt has founded, directed and partnered with several innovative companies. Most notably, in 2003 he invented a revolutionary new line of sport supplements that he used exclusively with the professional teams and athletes he was working with. In 2009, Matt chose to commercialize these formulas and make them available to athletes worldwide. Matt was a founding partner and the product formulator at BioSteel Sports Nutrition, a manufacturer and distributor of nutritional sports supplements. During his tenure with the company, he helped BioSteel grow from a start-up with a shoestring budget to a multi-million-dollar business with international distribution.

Matt and I have known each other for decades. Soon after we first met, he was chosen as the head strength and conditioning coach for

271

the Toronto Maple Leafs. I believe there is no other person with Matt's level of understanding of exceptional human movement and how to enhance it.

If you think back to the early days of your career, what skills or attributes do you think helped you shift your career so successfully?

My mom was a big influence on me, and she was one of these almost annoyingly optimistic people. She had the idea that things would always work out. Like that meme going around of the dog drinking coffee as a house burns down around him—that is how I was raised. "Everything is going to be okay. Everything is going to be fine. Just stay positive." The harsh reality of the world is that it is not always fine. Sometimes it just sucks, and it is shitty.

If I go back to 12 years ago, I was on top of the world with this high-profile job [strength and conditioning coach for the Toronto Maple Leafs], and I got fired. That could have been devastating or humiliating, but I was optimistic enough that I never equated my worth or my ability to my job title. I did not think I was any more special a person when I had a cool job title than I was before I had it. When it was gone, I still felt the same. I have always had a fairly strong work ethic. I may not always do things the best way, or the smartest way, or the most efficient way, but I am able to put my head down and do the work. The one thing I cling to now is that resilience and adaptability, especially in times like this pandemic. We were just talking about this pandemic and how our businesses are suffering, and no one knows when this will be over, but I do know that I am adaptable and resilient enough to make it through. I am optimistic enough to think that I do not know what normal even looks like right now, so there is no point worrying about that.

In the book there is a chapter dedicated to instinctual human movement (chapter 13). What do you think are the most important movement patterns that humans need to pay attention to?

The basics, regardless of your sport or your goals, are the things we were designed to be able to do: squat, lunge, push, pull, walk, run and jump. These are all things we probably had to do to survive to make it here. I know that in my training with athletes, we can sometimes become so fixated on the anatomy and biomechanics at such a high level, like some of the things you do as a chiropractor. We are working with special populations of people, from elite CEOs, business icons and then all the way over to the elite athletes. Sometimes we can be distracted by the latest, greatest, highly specific movement, then figuring out "How do we isolate this muscle?" So much of what we do in our training is track-and-field-type exercises. When you watch athletes do these activities, skipping and bounding and moving, you see them come alive.

I know that for myself I can feel awful on any given day and at six in the morning I am struggling to get out of bed, and then I get out on a field and I start to skip and bound, and suddenly I feel my body start to come alive. I can do things in that moment that I did not think I could do. Unfortunately, and especially now when we are forced to work out in confined spaces, we do not get to experience many of the movements we should, because we were designed to move in wide open spaces. To run and skip and jump. To change direction, to change levels and play. All the things we did regularly as kids. That aspect of play and dynamic movement, walking outside in nature on variable terrain, that is something that is particularly important on a basic human, fundamental level.

Was there a time in your life when facts or people were telling you to do something a certain way, or go in a certain direction in your life, but your instincts were telling you the opposite? What did you do, and how did things turn out?

That is the story of my entire life. All of my friends were hockey players, and I had no interest in playing hockey. I wanted to play football. I am from Waterloo, Ontario, within walking distance to two fantastic universities that I grew up spending tons of time at, swimming and playing basketball at Laurier then lifting weights and training at Waterloo. But I wanted to go to McGill and get out of town. I moved to Toronto on a whim, invited by a friend who helped me get a job, but I moved here with no plan, no contacts, and decided, after doing my undergraduate degree and then another degree at teachers' college, to scrap all that. I became a personal trainer in Toronto. My whole life has gone that way. Even when I invented a sugar-free sports drink [BioSteel], when every single nutritionist and dietician, basically every nutrition expert with a degree behind their name, told me I was crazy and that it could never be done, the research did not make sense and the ingredients would not work together. I could also tell you quite a few stories of where I followed my gut and things did not work out and I made stupid decisions. There is a long list of stupid ones to go with the success stories, but for the most part I have lived my life in an instinctual way, and it has worked out more often than not.

Do you think our instincts are related to our motivation? What do you see as the major drivers of behaviour in the athletes you work with?

Most of the athletes I am working with are considered elite—whether that is professional, amateur or Olympic level. Obviously, most of them are extremely hard-working. Some of them have done everything right, and turned over every stone in their preparation. But even that group is genetically blessed. It is a nice idea that the average person could accomplish some of these things through hard work, and that part matters, but winning the genetic lottery matters a ton too. Human beings tend to gravitate toward things and activities that bring them success. Why wouldn't you? If you are a really tall kid, you will probably gravitate toward volleyball or basketball because you will have way more success than you might have at gymnastics. If you are really fast, you will probably gravitate toward track and field. That regular experience of success is a factor. Then beyond that, at the NHL level, everyone has good genetics, and even a lazy NHL player probably works harder at training compared to the average person.

Then you can think about what drives the athletes at that level. For some people it is the fame. When you go out on the ice or the field, and you score a goal or a touchdown, and everyone is screaming your name and everyone is happy—some people are hooked on that feedback loop of using their athletic prowess to receive admiration, praise and love. For some people it is the social status and the notoriety. For some it is purely financial. Sometimes that motivation gets painted in a terribly negative light, but you need to understand that I have trained some athletes who come from horribly unfortunate circumstances growing up as kids, such as not knowing where your next meal is coming from or when you might eat again. Being forced to sleep on the floor. The financial drive that comes from that is a real thing. They can suddenly make life-changing amounts of money and even money that impacts their family for generations.

For most of the professional athletes, when you think about the instinctual motivation, they do have a drive to use their body in the best way possible, and they do find that by doing that, it makes them feel good. By doing what feels good, they can receive praise and adulation for their talents. It results in so much positive feedback, and the system supports what they love to do.

Our instincts to survive are some of the most powerful drivers of human behaviour. When you are watching your athletes in a competitive situation, do you think survival instincts play a role in their performance?

I think they feel that every single day they get an opportunity to score points, and that is what they like to do, even on an instinctual level. That is the one really cool thing about sports, but it can also be very stressful, because every day you are being scrutinized. There are not many jobs out there where your workday is on video and replayed constantly until the next time you are in the arena. Every single day, an athlete is being evaluated on everything they do. Can you imagine, in a normal workplace, if that was the case? Someone watching you while you are sitting at your computer working and evaluating every call you made, every email you sent, every report you wrote? Did you do it well? And, primarily, what did you not do well? I think for many athletes they enjoy the scoring and evaluation, and then it becomes a fight against nature to see how long you can sustain your performance or keep improving.

If you watch my athletes in the summer, sometimes when we are just playing tag for fun, they are dying to win that game. It has nothing to do with money, it has nothing to do with who is watching, it is a natural drive to be out there competing and seeing where you stack up. It makes sense when you think about this from an instinctual level. That is how we got here. At some point in time, you got up in the morning and you had to fight or compete. You had to fight to find something to eat and you had to fight to not be eaten by something else. It was humans versus whatever else was out there coming to get us. I think that feeling of competition and wanting to win is part of our instinctual drive. If you were talking to an anthropologist, they might describe a whole bunch of competitions and at some point humans won, and that is why we are here today. We are left with that internal drive to compete. It is always there.

You are what most people would call a "high-performer" in every sense of the word, but you are also very aware of the negative impacts that can have on your physical and mental well-being. What are your strategies for your personal wellness, mental health and fitness into this next year and beyond?

This is an extremely hard thing for me. It is something that I have had to work on, and I am still constantly working on. I am not as successful as I would like to be that way. I feel truly blessed because I absolutely love what I do, and I found a way to monetize it and get paid for it, but really, I was doing this before I ever got paid, and even if I was not able to get paid, I would try to keep doing it with anyone who would let me coach them. I feel that it is my purpose. That is when I feel happiest and most content. The problem with those types of feelings is that I cannot shut it off. I cannot leave the office and flick the lights off and not think about it until the next day. It just does not work for me.

I have tried many different forms of mindfulness and meditation. Most of them have not worked for me. A few years ago a friend gave me a book by Thich Nhat Hanh called *Peace Is Every Step*, and doing walking meditations has really hit home for me. That is something that I try to do more of, and I try to be in nature when I can. Usually, you would expect me to describe all the books I am reading, all the great titles for self-help, and I do that, but I also think it is important to have some junk food for my brain where I can just find something that is funny or stupid, whether it is a television show or a movie. I always have two books on my bedside table. One is educational—physiology, anatomy, biomechanics or even business-related—and the other one is a biography or story about educational characters that has absolutely nothing to do with my job, but it allows me to shut my brain off and go somewhere else before bedtime.

Every year around Christmas, my wife and I will sit down and do some puzzles. Usually, we are up north and having some quiet time.

This year we had way more time to work through our puzzles, and I found it more profound. The puzzle had more meaning for me this year. Number one, as soon as I got focused on the puzzle, I had to shut off everything else—my phone, my television—and forget about any other distractions. I was completely transfixed on this picture of my dog, basically a completely irrelevant project that has nothing to do with anything. It totally captured my attention. Unlike doing my bookkeeping and accounting—it could never do that!

People like me who are the leaders in our business are expected to be the ones with the answers. We are there to lead and provide solutions to the massive problems created within this pandemic. We are stuck in a period in history right now where there do not seem to be very many clear solutions to our problem, and even the mechanisms by which you would normally make a decision to solve a problem are not clear. I go back to those thoughts and I think, "Okay, it is no different than this massive jigsaw puzzle that I am working on."

I have to start by clearing away my workspace, making sure I have all the pieces available. Then I start with the borders because I know what those are. It seems impossible at the start, and I do not know how I will ever solve the whole thing, but I know the corner. I am good there; I do not know what that will lead to, but I can start somewhere. Then I can break things into sub-groups or sub-problems, and I will work on those. Some days you are convinced that there are pieces missing or that the manufacturer screwed up. Maybe you need to take a break. Then, on another day, a different part becomes clear. It was a great metaphor for my life, and believe it or not, it turned out to be an effective meditation tool for me.

—

Lynda
Reeves

*Your imagination gives
you the vision and something to
reach for, and then your
instincts tell you how to achieve it.*

LYNDA REEVES

LYNDA REEVES is the founder of *House & Home* magazine and its French-language counterpart, *Maison & Demeure*. Lynda has spent the past 30 years as a TV host and journalist, writing columns and speaking about design and decorating on national TV and radio. Over the years, Lynda and her team have designed and decorated many projects for great causes, including six of the grand prize show homes in support of the Princess Margaret Hospital Foundation for cancer research. Lynda mentors talented young designers through her own design firm, Lynda Reeves Design Studio. She lives in Toronto with her husband, travels frequently, and loves to cook and entertain. Lynda spends weekends at a lakehouse in northern Ontario—the subject of a ten-part series airing on *House & Home*'s website and its YouTube channel.

I am proud to be able to also refer to Lynda as a friend and a mentor for the past decade. Her enthusiasm and work ethic are something I am in awe of every time we talk. My major take-away related to instincts is as follows: To become someone who is an iconic thinker, you must have an imagination. Then you need to develop the confidence to trust your instincts and bring what you imagined to life.

Do you think our human instincts have an influence on how we design our homes, or how we set up our living spaces?

Totally. If you separate yourself from your rational knowledge, what the trends are and what everyone is telling you about how things should be, and instead you listen to how *you* feel, or what *you* are experiencing or even your own sensibility, then you start to make decisions based on a whole different set of criteria. The decisions usually come more easily, and if you don't second-guess yourself and you try to stop worrying about everything and asking all your friends what they think, *you* can usually make good decisions. If you do take a poll on these decisions or seek professional advice, you will find that often you come back to your first instincts.

Do people need to have more confidence to be able to rely on their instincts when designing a home?

Of course! It is all about that. I am *very* lucky that at this stage of my career, after doing this for over 35 or 40 years, I trust my instincts. That makes the decisions much quicker. Sometimes, after you make a decision, you might work through the logic and realize there is something you had not considered that forces you to have to take a different approach. But when it comes to things like colour, or a feeling that you want the place to have, or the priorities—instinctually you know! You know how you want to live. You know how you entertain; you know what things make you happy.

When you are scouting houses for the magazine, do you have an instinctual feeling about a location when you first walk in the door? What does that experience feel like?

The first thing is the instinct. Immediately! I am asking myself, "How does this house feel and how do I feel in this house?" I listen to myself.

If I feel a sense of awe, if I feel joy, if I feel excitement, if I feel elation—that is a winner. I know those feelings are not just unique to me; that is how most people will feel when they see this house or when they walk in. That is the first immediate instinct that kicks in. It has to do with trusting that if I am excited, you will be excited. Number two is figuring out how it will photograph. Can we capture this location to elicit these same feelings in a reader? That understanding comes from the experience of shooting so many houses and locations. The third thing is the backstory of the people who live there and the designer and how this all came to be. That decision relies on instinct also. If that story is interesting to me, it will be interesting to other people. There is so much being written now about bringing joy to your spaces, but ultimately you are talking about making *you* feel better! If I walk into a house and I feel excited and happy, they have done something right. They have listened to their instincts. The emotion of the homeowner and/or the designer will come through when they have listened to their instincts.

Our bestselling covers are not the most beautiful rooms. Our bestselling covers are pictures like the one with two little kids on their way to the barn with their chickens. The covers that strike a chord are the ones that say something about the humans living there, and the ones that give you a feeling that you want to capture in your own life.

You have been able to work with, observe and interview some of the top designers in the world. We would probably both agree that these iconic people listen to their inner instincts in their design work, but do you think there is something more that allows them to rise to the level of "Iconic Designer"?

If we are thinking about our generation, the single most influential designer of homes and interiors was Ralph Lauren. He influenced so many great people. If you think of many of the homes featured in movies such as *Something's Gotta Give* and many similar movies directed by Nancy Meyers, his design had a significant influence on that sensibility. He was the first person of our generation to understand that a room tells a story. He started out looking for backdrops for his fashion photography and spaces for his models. He was designing clothes that were romantic and then safari, and many of the shoots started out in old English country houses, but eventually he needed an American version that was fresh and exciting, but also full of drama and told a story. That is when he came up with his interior design collection.

Ralph Lauren is more of a stylist and less of a designer. In his mind, he was creating a setting for these women and men to lounge around that would make us want their lifestyle, and then ultimately want to buy the clothes. He was brilliant! It all happened because he had a great, vivid imagination. He also had confidence to try something new, like putting a guy in a polo outfit in an elaborate drawing room with silver candelabras. He knew this was complete fantasy, and people just ate it up. Then it just kept going from there. He did the ski chalet, and the lodge, and the ranch in Aspen, and it just kept going for so many years. I would say, based on the success of his design influence, the most important things for this iconic success are: you have to have an imagination, and you have to use that imagination to tell a story that people want—something that we believe could be attainable and something we want to aspire to.

We all thought those Ralph Lauren rooms could be attainable. When he did the mansion in New York, I will never forget the first time I walked into those rooms. My pulse would quicken. He knew how to adjust the scale and the fabrics to make everything feel luxurious. The attention to detail was extreme, right down to the forks on the tables, the colours were beautiful, and we had never seen that before. I believe he used his instincts and his imagination to create something iconic and amazing. I think your imagination gives you the vision and something to reach for, and then your instincts tell you how to achieve it, and you need to trust that.

Dave Salmoni

An animal believes, on an instinctual level, "if you are good to me, I will be good to you." That connection can make you feel part of something bigger.

DAVE SALMONI

DAVE SALMONI is one of Canada's best-known animal experts and has helped people throughout the world gain a better understanding of many species of animals through his extensive work in television. Dave studied zoology at Laurentian University and wrote his undergraduate thesis on tracking the hibernation of black bears. Also while in university, he was certified in Biological Immobilization of Wildlife.

One of the interesting things we talk about in this interview is Dave's incredible work teaching captive-born tigers how to hunt, kill and eventually live wild at the Tiger Moon Sanctuary in South Africa. This exciting process was documented in Discovery Channel's *Living with Tigers* (2003).

Today, Dave works in television production and is a regular guest with his furry and feathered friends on *Jimmy Kimmel*. I was interested in talking with Dave about the similarities and differences between animal instincts and human instincts. This interview was incredibly enlightening and I now have an even deeper love for animals and nature. One of the most important things that Dave was able to help me understand is the difference between just "acting" on our instincts, as animals do, and "understanding" our instincts. This is what humans *should* do, because we can.

Can you tell me a bit about the journey of your life that led you to the work you do now? From the outside, it looks incredibly exciting and fun, but it is also such a unique area of work.

The arc of the story starts with being an animal lover. Even back when I was in grade one, I told my mom I wanted to be a zoologist. I was never one to conform. I did not like authority, and I still do not—just ask my wife. [Laughs.] Because of that, my grades were always mediocre. I just did what I had to and tried to keep everyone off my back.

In high school, I realized that I wanted to be able to go away and be with the animals, because that was what I loved. I went on to do my first university degree in zoology and then everyone said, well, you should probably continue to a doctorate degree, because at that time that is what everyone did. But it did not really work for me, because the better you were in my field academically, the more you were forced into the lab to work, and the less time you had to be with and experience the animals, compared with my undergraduate, where I was able to spend almost my entire fourth year tracking black bears. I was watching the bears and also bumping into moose, watching elk. For me, that was the dream.

I then began to apply to work at the local zoos, and a smaller, privately owned zoo brought me on. This group really believed in the concept of preventing animal boredom. The owner wanted every animal to be able to come out of their cage and play. My job was to find out what they liked to do, and make sure they got to do it all day. I fully bought in to this idea, I loved it, and I moved there. This led to me becoming an animal trainer, because so much of the work I was doing at the zoo was basically that.

I had an interesting experience only two days in that pushed me toward my love of big cats. I then became the main trainer for the big cats, but after a while I sort of fell out of love with the zoo industry.

I transferred into more feature film and production type of work. After that, a conservation job came up within ecotourism where a tiger sanctuary was being planned in South Africa. They decided to use captive tigers and release them into the sanctuary, and my job then became teaching these tigers to hunt. When the world told me that this could not be done, I responded with a greater determination to get this done.

It took me five years living with those tigers, and at the end of it the tigers were hunting by themselves, and that experience was my first main exposure to television. This type of programming, probably thanks to Steve Irwin, was extremely popular at this time. I would finish one project and then they would ask me, "What do you want to do next?" I wanted to live with a pride of lions, so I went to do that. Then it became sharks, then bears, and that continued for ten years. Basically, I would have a question in my head about a certain animal and through television I was able to explore that and make a living doing it.

You were living a life that many of us would be very envious of!

I think it would seem like that, but remember, I also had to sleep in a tent for about five years; I was chased around the world by mercenary soldiers; I had spinal surgery. At least once a year, something almost killed me! People want my job when the tigers are just lying back and relaxing or licking my face. Of course, those days are awesome—but it is when that big male lion wants to eat you that things change. I do not look back on it and think of the negative things, but I could tell you enough stories that would make you not want my job.

What does the concept of instinct mean to you?

My scientific brain would just go to the basic definition of it: instincts are inherent behaviours that do not require much thought. In general, instincts can be something you are born with, and I think it is an impulse to a behaviour and it can then manifest itself in those behaviours—or not, depending on how you use your brain.

I think that wild animals are honed to their instinct because it allows them to survive. Domesticated animals have instincts, but we refer to them as muted, due to the domestication. Then the next state of removal is humans, because our intellect gets in the way. If an instinct is supposed to be a thoughtless behaviour, then we might look at that as a Neanderthal behaviour, and maybe think that we should not do that.

Our instincts exist, it is just a matter of someone cutting through the weeds a bit to say, "This is what your instinct is." Then we can get into some of the bigger behaviours, such as things that we are attracted to or situations that would cause us to become aggressive. In a social setting, you might think that you are using your brain to decide that someone is being a jerk, but I think we could prove that your thought process is probably more instinctual, and that is an example of your instincts kicking in.

The most common version of instincts in humans is more about personality traits—things like Type A personality, or a more submissive, quiet personality, people who are drawn to a life of data crunching and the various personalities that we put into these larger groupings. Those personalities were not chosen; you were born with them. You then developed them, and you found comfort in them and therefore became them. Becoming what we call a Type A personality is not something you consciously choose; I think you are born that way and that your instincts have a role in that. Instincts like this exist in all humans, they are just not as obvious as when I am teaching a tiger to hunt. This is true of all behaviour in the world. The instinct is there somewhere.

When you think about connecting with animals and nature, what things do you think we could improve that would benefit us as a society?

You could analyze this from a literal view and say that altruism is something that we are born with and having a connection to something then feeds into our altruistic instincts. I believe 100 percent that the world would be better off if we were more connected to animals and nature. This is basically a big part of what I do for a living.

When we talk about the *Jimmy Kimmel* clips where I bring various animals on his show, the only reason I go out there is not for the money, and not to be famous, but because Jimmy's audience is not the audience that I already have from the regular work I do in wildlife. If you are already into wildlife, you have probably already watched some of my other films. I go to *Jimmy Kimmel* because I have a chance to connect with millions of people whom I may not otherwise reach. I can explain to them how awesome it is to connect with other creatures on this planet. This is important because we know that, once you are connected to them, you see their value. Once you feel or see their value, then you become more of a conservationist. The value for humanity is to find that connection.

I think that, on a basic level, it is proven that children who grow up around animals will have more empathy, and with empathy you will become a better person with a better sense of your surroundings, along with an advanced understanding of how other people operate. Interestingly, we find that a lot of "loners" in society are really attracted to animals. This is because, if you are not clued in to regular social ideals that make you popular or accepted, an animal does not care about any of that. It makes sense because an animal believes, on an instinctual level, "if you are good to me, I will be good to you." Animals can see through all the social "crud" to know that your heart is in the right place, and once that connection is made, you do feel more self-worth due to the mutual admiration. That connection can make you feel part of something bigger, it makes you feel special, all those things that make you feel healthier. If you need a connection, go rescue a dog, or if you are that person who is a bit of a loner and you prefer data crunching to humans, maybe try to spend more time with animals.

I have noticed things in my life, for example swimming in a lake or walking with my dog, that instantly improve my mood and my overall feeling of well-being. Do you have similar examples in your life, when nature positively affected your mood?

Yes! I think these things are what we would refer to as "triggers." For example, whenever I go camping, I am anxious to sweep up my campsite. My wife always laughs at me because I *never* do this much sweeping at home. The reason I immediately want to sweep the campsite, remove all the small rocks and pine needles, is because I cannot wait to get my shoes off! I love the feeling of walking around outdoors with no shoes. It relaxes me and, in a way, it is a trigger for me.

I think that people who are more "in tune" with their instincts are more aware of these positive triggers and how they can improve their mood. This is where instincts and behaviour can overlap. When we talk about the bond between humans and animals, if you have realized that connection, it is such a source of those positive feelings. It is rare for your dog or cat or whatever to trigger a stress feeling. The animals and your connection, for those of us who value those bonds with our animals, can become a constant source of those positive feelings.

Do you have an example where you followed your instincts, even though the facts or other people were pointing you in another direction, but in the end following your instincts was the right way to go?

The best example of instincts for me is the thing that people know me most for, the unique path that my life has taken. I have been lucky enough to be filled with passion, and I know it is a cliché word, but I believe that many people do not actually get to "feel" it on a regular basis. In my case, because I am such an instinctual human being, almost always and at every turn, intellect would tell me, "Don't do that!"

I would say that the number one instinctive drive for me has always been related to my self-confidence and my own self-reliance, in both good and bad situations. Sometimes it can make you seem like an arrogant jerk, but it can also guide you through a lot of trouble. If you really want something in your life, particularly if you are chasing a passion, you will often need to make some uncomfortable decisions. Everything that turned out to be "uniquely" passion-driven in my life was successful because of my instincts. I never spent hours thinking these things through in an intellectual framework. I somehow managed it in my own brain, had my own confidence and created the path. Even in many situations with lions or big cats when I had to put my life on the line, sometimes being charged by them 30 times a day, in my head my instincts told me, "I can do this."

FINAL THOUGHTS
ON INSTINCTS

- We are instinctually attracted to things (or people) that are like us, and we are often instinctually unsure about things (or people) that are different from us. This instinct requires us to acknowledge this attraction and then use our cognitive skills to think through what is real and how we should act. For example, if someone looks quite different from you, your instincts could elicit an uneasy feeling about interacting with them, but that feeling is not an accurate understanding of the potential relationship you could have with this person. You will feel better acknowledging these feelings and then using your cognitive analysis and learned experience to make an accurate assessment of the situation or person.

- We instinctually like to compete and play games. These activities allow us to release emotions and expend energy in a way that is healthy for both our physical and mental well-being. This instinct can be applied to many areas of our life—work, community and even our family situations. If you turn something that is challenging or maybe boring into a game, suddenly you will grab everyone's attention. We also tend to enjoy being physically active more when there is a game involved, as opposed to expending energy for no particular reason.

- The instincts for attachment and connection are the most important pathways for normal human development and maturation.
We should try to structure our lives to honour these instincts
through our rituals and our time spent connecting with others. It
is extremely important that we allow time for this space and freedom within our relationships. That way, we will be able to honour
and develop these instincts to their full potential.

- Humans have an instinctual relationship to food and the energy it
provides. We will be healthier, more productive and even more satisfied when we take the time to understand and appreciate where
our food comes from and how we prepare it. We benefit from eating in an instinctual way because it improves our clarity about the
value of good nutrition and our overall enjoyment of the experience.

- We have instincts that allow us to be curious and creative. When
we spend time and energy following these instincts, we will add
more joy and passion to our lives.

- Our brains and our bodies were instinctually designed to be moving regularly, and ideally outside in nature, every day. These
experiences have benefits that are both physiological and emotional. If that movement serves a purpose, for example walking
our dog or going on a hike with friends, we seem to enjoy it even
more and the benefits are greater.

- Blindly following something or someone is, in most cases, a bad
idea. We should get rid of the saying "follow your instincts" and
replace it with "understand your instincts" or even "honour your
instincts." Our instincts are incredibly powerful and important,
but they also have potential to cause us harm or lead us toward
bad decisions. If we take the time and make the effort to combine our instincts with our intelligence and experience, we can
then find our best potential. We will discover our ability to turn
instincts into human superpowers.

ACKNOWLEDGEMENTS

I WHOLEHEARTEDLY BELIEVE that the best things in life are accomplished when you are part of a great team that works well together. I have been extremely fortunate during my experience writing *Your Better Instincts* to have been propped up by some of the best teammates ever.

The accomplished group at Page Two has made the last couple of years always bearable and often enjoyable. During the extensive writing process, I repeatedly told friends and family how privileged I felt to be able to find the time and support to write a book. Without the steadfast and experienced guidance of this team, it would not have been possible.

Special thanks to Trena White for her initial interest in my many ideas about human instincts, and for pairing me with the most brilliant editor, Amanda Lewis. I honestly believe that Amanda is my long-lost nature-loving "soul mate." Throughout the writing process, she truly "got me" and understood what I was trying to say—even if I did not always articulate it very well. Amanda's magical talent of turning my words into something much more impactful and understandable was the best gift ever. Other notable members of the Page Two team were copy editor John Sweet; project managers Caela Moffet and Elana Dublanko, who together kept us all organized and running on track (not easy!); proofreader Alison Strobel; designer Taysia Louie; and Meghan O'Neill in marketing.

I have immense love and gratitude for my husband, Tim, and my children Matthew, Estella and Jackson, who consistently helped me find perspective and motivation to live with the ideas and concepts presented in this book. They worked incredibly hard to give me the space and time I needed to write and think. Tim took many hours out of jam-packed workdays to read sections of the book and provide both helpful and practical feedback. There were sacrifices made as we tried to juggle our busy sports and school schedules. Tim would help me figure out ways to escape to a quiet corner (anywhere) to try to finish another few pages of writing. My family's enthusiasm about my topic and the interview subjects gave me the stamina to keep moving forward... even during a pandemic where, as small business owners, we experienced some incredibly dark days along with motivational challenges.

Speaking of inspiration in dark times, the incredible group of people who agreed to help me out with the interview section of the book provided amazing insight and respite from the extensive monotony of lockdown. I had pictured a much different format when we originally planned this part of the book and how the interviews would play out, but, like many things over this past year, we adapted. A few of the interviews were completed in person, but soon, due to increasing restrictions, Zoom became the technology of choice. I appreciate all the wisdom they shared with me and that they took the time out of their incredibly busy lives to answer all my questions with enthusiasm and thoughtfulness. Huge thanks to Stephen Grant, Chris Hadfield, Geddy Lee, Alex Lifeson, Dr. Deborah MacNamara, Tracy Moore, Matt Nichol, Lynda Reeves and Dave Salmoni. Your incredible insight and ideas will resonate with me always.

NOTES

Introduction

It was a world of waste and wonder ... Quotations from the published book:
Tomos Roberts and Nocomo (Illus.), *The Great Realization* (New York:
HarperCollins, 2020). The video: *The Great Realisation*, Probably
Tomfoolery, April 29, 2020, YouTube, 4:00, youtube.com/watch?v=
Nw5KQMXDiM4.

Chapter 1: Why Instincts?

18th-century novelist Jean Paul ... "Jean Paul," *Encyclopedia Britannica*, britan
nica.com/biography/Jean-Paul.
average life expectancy in Canada ... Tracey Bushnik, Michael Tjepkema and
Laurent Martel, "Health-Adjusted Life Expectancy in Canada," Statistics
Canada, www150.statcan.gc.ca/n1/pub/82-003-x/2018004/article/54950-
eng.htm; "Gap in Life Expectancy Projected to Decrease between Aboriginal
People and the Total Canadian Population," Statistics Canada, www150.
statcan.gc.ca/n1/pub/89-645-x/2010001/life-expectancy-esperance-vie-
eng.htm.
In the United States, life expectancy has declined ... National Center for Health
Statistics, "Life Expectancy," Centers for Disease Control and Prevention,
cdc.gov/nchs/fastats/life-expectancy.htm.

experts have given our youth a mark of D... "Family Influence: The 2020
ParticipACTION Report Card on Physical Activity for Children and Youth,"
ParticipACTION, participaction.com/en-ca/resources/children-and-youth-
report-card.

Chapter 3: Understanding Our Instincts

Malcolm Gladwell talks extensively about this concept... Malcolm Gladwell,
Blink: The Power of Thinking without Thinking (New York: Back Bay Books,
2005).
Pavlov was a Nobel Prize–winning scientist... Kendra Cherry, "Ivan Pavlov
and His Discovery of Classical Conditioning," Verywell Mind, March 27,
2020, verywellmind.com/ivan-pavlov-biography-1849-1936-2795548#:~:
text=Ivan%20Pavlov%20was%20a%20Russian,upon%20the%20
presentation%20of%20food.
INSTINCT—Is the inherent disposition... "Reference Terms: Instinct,"
ScienceDaily, sciencedaily.com/terms/instinct.htm#:~:text=Instinct%20
is%20the%20inherent%20disposition,broad%20spectrum%20of%20
animal%20life.
One of my favourite definitions... *Merriam-Webster*, s.v. "instinct," merriam-
webster.com/dictionary/instinct.
How do migratory birds, herding dogs, and navigating sea turtles... Mark S.
Blumberg, "Development Evolving: The Origins and Meanings of Instinct,"
WIRES Cognitive Science 8, nos. 1–2 (January 2017), doi.org/10.1002/wcs.1371.

Chapter 5: Modern Life and Its Impact on Our Instincts

surveys designed to evaluate the new gig economy... Susan J. Ashford, Brianna
Barker Caza and Erin M. Reid, "From Surviving to Thriving in the Gig
Economy: A Research Agenda for Individuals in the New World of
Work," *Research in Organizational Behavior* 38 (2018), doi.org/10.1016/j.
riob.2018.11.001.

a famous study by Jeremy Morris... J.N. Morris et al., "Coronary Heart-
Disease and Physical Inactivity of Work," *Lancet* 262, no. 6798 (1953),
doi.org/10.1016/S0140-6736(53)91495-0.

one in three adolescents aged 13 to 18 will experience an anxiety disorder...
Stats in this section as cited in Amy Ellis Nutt, "Why Kids and Teens
May Face Far More Anxiety These Days," *Washington Post*, May 10,
2018, washingtonpost.com/news/to-your-health/wp/2018/05/10/
why-kids-and-teens-may-face-far-more-anxiety-these-days/.

research overwhelmingly supports the concept of free play... See several articles
on Active for Life, activeforlife.com/multisportadvantage/.

Chapter 6: Instincts to Survive—Human Evolution— Then and Now

Yuval Noah Harari, in his recent book... Yuval Noah Harari, *Sapiens: A Brief
History of Humankind* (New York: HarperCollins, 2014).

The earliest groups of Homo sapiens... Christopher S. Henshilwood and Curtis
W. Marean, "The Origin of Modern Human Behavior: Critique of the Models
and Their Test Implications," *Current Anthropology* 44, no. 5 (2003),
doi.org/10.1086/377665.

Chapter 7: Instincts for Animal Connection

positive benefits of relationships between animals and humans... "About Pets &
People," Centers for Disease Control and Prevention, cdc.gov/healthypets/
health-benefits/index.html.

Chapter 8: Instincts for Human Connection

*based on the theory of evolution, procreation is always cited as the origin of the
original drive*... Phillip Sloan, "Darwin: From *Origin of Species* to *Descent of
Man*," Stanford Encyclopedia of Philosophy, June 17, 2019, plato.stanford.
edu/entries/origin-descent/.

Harvard Study of Adult Development began in 1938... "Harvard Study of Adult Development," Maelstrom Research (Research Institute of the McGill University Health Centre), maelstrom-research.org/mica/individual-study/hsad.

Donn Byrne was most famous for his theories on similarity and attraction... Donn Byrne, "An Overview (and Underview) of Research and Theory within the Attraction Paradigm," *Journal of Social and Personal Relationships* 14, no. 3 (1997), doi.org/10.1177%2F0265407597143008.

the only significant determinant of attraction was similarity... As cited in Maria Airth, "Similarity-Attraction Paradigm: Definition & Criticisms," Study.com, study.com/academy/lesson/similarity-attraction-paradigm-definition-criticisms.html.

Mirroring, also called isopraxism, is essentially imitation... Chris Voss, *Never Split the Difference: Negotiating as if Your Life Depended on It* (New York: HarperCollins, 2016).

Chapter 9: Instincts and Family Life

An interesting study looked at the effects of oxytocin on mice... Bianca J. Marlin et al., "Oxytocin Enables Maternal Behaviour by Balancing Cortical Inhibition," *Nature* 520 (2015), doi.org/10.1038/nature14402.

Chapter 10: Instincts for Communication

a restricted developmental period during which the nervous system is particularly sensitive... Dale Purves et al., eds., *Neuroscience*, 2nd ed. (Sunderland, MA: Sinauer Associates, 2001).

in rare cases where children were not exposed to communication prior to puberty... Joshua K. Hartshorne, Joshua B. Tenenbaum and Steven Pinker, "A Critical Period for Second Language Acquisition: Evidence from 2/3 Million English Speakers," *Cognition* 177 (2018), doi.org/10.1016/j.cognition.2018.04.007.

A fascinating discovery that sheds light on this concept... Joyce W. Lacy and Craig E.L. Stark, "The Neuroscience of Memory: Implications for the Courtroom," *Nature Reviews Neuroscience* 14 (2013), doi.org/10.1038/nrn3563.

Chapter 11: Enhancing and Honouring Our Basic Instincts by Spending More Time in Nature

trees can communicate with each other... Peter Wohlleben, *The Hidden Life of Trees: What They Feel, How They Communicate—Discoveries from a Secret World* (Vancouver: Greystone Books, 2016).

the growing obesity crisis across North America... Stacy Irvine, "Using Exercise to Enhance Your Brain Power," *Huffington Post*, November 22, 2011, huffing tonpost.ca/stacy-irvine-dc-msc/exercise-your-brain-power_b_964448.html.

each of us seems to have a primal drive toward life... Harry J. Stead, "Why Long Walks Will Change Your Life," HarryJStead.co.uk, February 29, 2020, harryj stead.co.uk/essays/2020/2/29/why-long-walks-will-change-your-life.

a recent book by Florence Williams... Florence Williams, *The Nature Fix: Why Nature Makes Us Happier, Healthier, and More Creative* (New York: W.W. Norton, 2017).

incidence of ADHD and depression have been steadily growing... "Data and Statistics about ADHD," Centers for Disease Control and Prevention, cdc.gov/NCBDDD/adhd/data.html.

changes in our body after only 20 minutes in nature... MaryCarol R. Hunter, Brenda W. Gillespie and Sophie Yu-Pu Chen, "Urban Nature Experiences Reduce Stress in the Context of Daily Life Based on Salivary Biomarkers," *Frontiers in Psychology* 10, art. no. 722 (2019), doi.org/10.3389/fpsyg.2019.00722.

Chapter 12: Instincts for Recovery and Rest

the best way for your body to physically and emotionally be able to recover... Courtney Connley, "LeBron James Reveals the Nighttime Routine That Helps Him Perform 'at the Highest Level,'" CNBC, December 23, 2018, cnbc.com/2018/12/21/lebron-james-reveals-the-nighttime-routine-that-sets-him-up-for-success.html.

Sleep is recorded in several stages... Eric Suni, "Stages of Sleep," Sleep Foundation, August 14, 2020, sleepfoundation.org/how-sleep-works/stages-of-sleep. This article includes links to several relevant sleep studies.

The CDC has listed airline attendants' work schedules as a risk factor... National Institute for Occupational Safety and Health, "Aircrew Safety & Health," Centers for Disease Control and Prevention, cdc.gov/niosh/topics/aircrew/cancer.html.

the causal relationship between sleep disruption and increased incidence of various cancers... Hye-Eun Lee et al., "The Relationship between Night Work and Breast Cancer," *Annals of Occupational and Environmental Medicine* 30, no. 1 (2018), doi.org/10.1186/s40557-018-0221-4.

Lack of sleep is linked to depression, cancer, obesity, cardiovascular disease... Goran Medic, Micheline Wille and Michiel E.H. Hemels, "Short- and Long-Term Health Consequences of Sleep Disruption," *Nature and Science of Sleep* 9 (2017), doi.org/10.2147/NSS.S134864.

Chapter 13: Instincts and Physical Performance

Humans have evolved from walking up to roughly 16 kilometres... James O'Keefe et al., "Achieving Hunter-Gatherer Fitness in the 21st Century: Back to the Future," *American Journal of Medicine* 123, no. 12 (2010), doi.org/10.1016/j.amjmed.2010.04.026; Thom Rieck, "10,000 Steps a Day: Too Low? Too High?" Mayo Clinic, March 23, 2020, mayoclinic.org/healthy-lifestyle/fitness/in-depth/10000-steps/art-20317391.

A large-scale study in Finland evaluated 2,613 elite male athletes... Jonatan R. Ruiz et al., "Strenuous Endurance Exercise Improves Life Expectancy: It's in Our Genes," *British Journal of Sports Medicine* 45, no. 3 (2011), doi.org/10.1136/bjsm.2010.075085.

A large-scale study utilizing data from mobile devices... Neil Savage, "Mobile Data: Made to Measure," *Nature* 527 (2015), doi.org/10.1038/527S12a.

study published in the Journal of the American College of Cardiology *evaluated 138 novice runners*... Anish N. Bhuva et al., "Training for a First-Time Marathon Reverses Age-Related Aortic Stiffening," *Journal of the American College of Cardiology* 75, no. 1 (2020), doi.org/10.1016/j.jacc.2019.10.045.

first documented athlete in this sphere was Eugen Sandow... "Eugen Sandow," *Encyclopedia Britannica*, britannica.com/biography/Eugen-Sandow.

Chapter 14: Instinctual Eating

The value of global food and agricultural production . . . Food and Agriculture
Organization of the United Nations, *Statistical Yearbook 2020* (Rome: FAO,
2020), fao.org/3/i3107e/i3107e01.pdf.

the manufacturers of processed food argue . . . Michael Moss, *Salt, Sugar, Fat:
How the Food Giants Hooked Us* (Toronto: Signal, 2013).

prevalence of worldwide obesity tripled between 1975 and 2016 . . . "Obesity and
Overweight," World Health Organization, April 1, 2020, who.int/news-room/
fact-sheets/detail/obesity-and-overweight.

Chapter 15: Once We Know Better . . . Then What?

meta-analysis of 26 studies related to implementation intentions . . . Ariane
Bélanger-Gravel, Gaston Godin and Steve Amireault, "A Meta-Analytic
Review of the Effect of Implementation Intentions on Physical Activity,"
Health Psychology Review 7, no. 1 (2013), doi.org/10.1080/17437199.2011.560
095.

Our genes do not eliminate the need for hard work . . . James Clear, *Atomic Habits:
An Easy & Proven Way to Build Good Habits & Break Bad Ones* (New York:
Avery, 2018).

Chapter 16: Summary of Our Human Instincts

An oft-quoted book on this subject . . . John Lubbock, *The Use of Life* (London:
Macmillan, 1894).

We are not enemies, but friends . . . Abraham Lincoln as quoted in Ronald C.
White Jr., *Lincoln's Greatest Speech: The Second Inaugural* (New York: Simon
& Schuster, 2002).

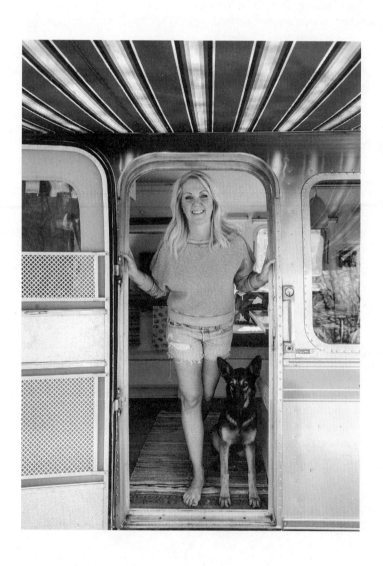

ABOUT THE AUTHOR

D R. STACY IRVINE has worked in the health and fitness industry for most of her life—first as a coach for many sports, where she was dedicated to training athletes competing for provincial and national teams throughout Saskatchewan, Manitoba and Ontario. Today, as the founder and co-owner of Totum Life Science, a national leader in the sports medicine, fitness and health care industry, with five locations in Toronto, Dr. Irvine also works regularly in Canadian and US media as a health and fitness expert for *Cityline* and *Breakfast Television* along with various print publications throughout Ontario and associated public speaking engagements. Dr. Irvine's formal education includes a bachelor's degree in kinesiology, a master's degree in exercise physiology and a doctorate of chiropractic. She has spent many years acquiring specialized training related to high-performance coaching and her clinical practice. Her patients and clientele range from absolute beginners just starting out on a health and fitness journey to elite young athletes, adult professional athletes and even a few celebrities. Dr. Irvine is an outdoor enthusiast. Her favourite place on earth is her Airstream trailer parked on a small private lake in the woods of Muskoka.

yourbetterinstincts.com
totum.ca